T0202081

Listening for What Matters

Listening for What Matters

Avoiding Contextual Errors in Health Care

SECOND EDITION ■

SAUL J. WEINER, MD
STAFF PHYSICIAN, JESSE BROWN VA MEDICAL CENTER
DEPUTY DIRECTOR, VA CENTER FOR INNOVATION IN
COMPLEX CHRONIC HEALTHCARE
PROFESSOR OF MEDICINE,
PEDIATRICS AND MEDICAL EDUCATION
UNIVERSITY OF ILLINOIS AT CHICAGO

AND

ALAN SCHWARTZ, PHD
THE MICHAEL REESE ENDOWED
PROFESSOR OF MEDICAL EDUCATION
RESEARCH PROFESSOR OF PEDIATRICS
UNIVERSITY OF ILLINOIS AT CHICAGO

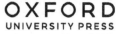

OXFORD
UNIVERSITY PRESS

OXFORD
UNIVERSITY PRESS

Oxford University Press is a department of the University of Oxford. It furthers the University's objective of excellence in research, scholarship, and education by publishing worldwide. Oxford is a registered trade mark of Oxford University Press in the UK and certain other countries.

Published in the United States of America by Oxford University Press
198 Madison Avenue, New York, NY 10016, United States of America.

Library of Congress Cataloging-in-Publication Data
Names: Weiner, Saul J. author. | Schwartz, Alan, 1970– author.
Title: Listening for what matters : avoiding contextual errors in health care /
Saul J. Weiner and Alan Schwartz.
Description: 2nd edition. | New York, NY : Oxford University Press, [2023] |
Includes bibliographical references and index. |
Identifiers: LCCN 2023011402 (print) | LCCN 2023011403 (ebook) |
ISBN 9780197588109 (paperback) | ISBN 9780197588116 (epub) | ISBN 9780197588130
Subjects: MESH: Physician-Patient Relations | Treatment Adherence and
Compliance | Attitude of Health Personnel | Patient Care Planning |
Patient-Centered Care | Medical Errors—prevention & control
Classification: LCC R729.8 (print) | LCC R729.8 (ebook) | NLM W 62 |
DDC 610.289—dc23/eng/20230515
LC record available at https://lccn.loc.gov/2023011402
LC ebook record available at https://lccn.loc.gov/2023011403

DOI: 10.1093/med/9780197588109.001.0001

Printed by Marquis Book Printing, Canada

CONTENTS

FOREWORD TO THE SECOND EDITION

The good physician treats the disease; the great physician treats the patient who has the disease.

—Sir William Osler (attributed)

A fundamental and enduring foundation of clinical care is the relationship between clinician and patient. Individuals seeking assistance share intimate details of their symptoms, fears, and concerns. The best clinicians, through the caring and the carefully formulated questions they ask, elicit the patient's story and integrate what they learn into their approach to the patient's care. Despite astonishing advances in medical technology including imaging, sophisticated blood tests, and the wide availability of medical information online and elsewhere, the patient's story remains essential to the clinical care enterprise. Drawing on that story to provide personalized care that considers each patient's unique situation, including their preferences and priorities, remains central to clinical expertise. How can we tell when we are doing it effectively or when there are substantial opportunities to improve?

We have learned a great deal from decades of research on physician–patient communication (e.g., how frequently and rapidly clinicians interrupt patients, the importance of patients' trust to their following recommendations to change their health behaviors). Multiple studies have applied a range of methods for analyzing conversations between clinicians and patients because a more narrow focus on strictly clinical data including test results, diagnoses, and treatment plans provides limited insight about why, how, and when individuals seek care and how clinical decisions are made.

The work of Drs. Weiner and Schwartz has focused on contextual cues that patients share during encounters with clinicians and their capacity to integrate what they learn about the life challenges their patients face as they collaboratively plan their care. Their studies have required direct observation of thousands of clinical encounters. They have been trailblazers in developing approaches, including the use of unannounced standardized patients and, more recently, enlisting willing patients to assist with audio-recording their visits. Their contributions have led to foundational insights about how attention to patient life context impacts a range of health-care priorities, including health-care outcomes and costs.

Weiner and Schwartz have not been satisfied (only) with impressive publications but have been equally passionate about testing practical approaches to incorporate into routine practice to improve care. For example, over the last decade physicians at nine Veterans Affairs medical centers and community clinics have enthusiastically participated in programs to improve attention to veteran life context in care planning, utilizing feedback from recordings of clinical encounters. They also engage trainees not only as research subjects but as junior colleagues, providing them with data and tools to draw their attention to veteran life context in the clinical setting—and opportunities to participate in quality improvement. The salutary impact of these programs on veterans' care, and on the clinicians who serve them, is documented in several studies described in this volume.

The importance of the broader context in which patients present as they seek care is hard to overstate. At this writing the United States and all countries have been struggling to respond to the emergence of an unprecedented pandemic which has both revealed in sharp relief and exacerbated preexisting fault lines in health-care delivery, including inequities in health and health care associated with race, ethnicity, income, education, geography, and more. Effective treatment of individuals with COVID-19 has required knowledge of patients' work, home situation, trust in medical information, and far more. A capacity to draw on that knowledge during clinical interactions has never been more vital to effective patient care.

The lessons of the pandemic will impact how and where care is provided as the threat of COVID-19 recedes, which should inspire both optimism and humility. While practice arrangements are likely to continue to evolve and may at times feel disruptive, understanding "the patient with the disease" will continue to be of enduring importance. The work of Drs. Weiner and Schwartz provides a framework for asking "Are we pursuing that understanding?"—and a set of tools for answering whether we are. Their work inspires both admiration and excitement and provides an opportunity to improve care through the thoughtful application of the findings and techniques described in *Listening for What Matters*.

Carolyn M. Clancy, MD, MACP
Department of Veterans Affairs
November 2022

FOREWORD TO THE FIRST EDITION

In the nostalgic days of Norman Rockwell, general practitioners practiced in small to medium-sized communities and had lifelong relationships with their patients. Some of these relationships and knowledge persist among primary care providers today, particularly those who have looked after their patients for many years. However, for many more patients, health care is fragmented, with multiple providers, short periods for direct physician interaction, and increasing complexity of patients' lives as they change jobs and move frequently. In the 2008 "great recession," we saw the way in which well-established individuals at many social class levels became unemployed.

What happens when doctors no longer understand how their patients' lives affect their health care? In their research into "contextualizing care," Saul Weiner and Alan Schwartz have tried to understand how and why physicians fail to incorporate patient context in care planning and how to more effectively deal with these failures. These contextual errors are medical errors—"failure of a planned action to be completed as intended or the use of the wrong plan to achieve an aim"[1]—and Schwartz and Weiner's studies demonstrate that they are widespread.

In tackling their challenge, they have created novel investigative and educational methodologies and have provided additional insights into the way in which physicians generally communicate with patients. Ten broad domains of patient context are identified, including access to care, social support, competing responsibilities, financial situation, relationship with health-care providers, skills and abilities, emotional state, cultural/spiritual beliefs, environment, and attitudes toward illness.

Weiner and Schwartz have focused their attention upon the most efficient and effective way for the busy physician to understand the context of the patient's life, so as to help with a sensible and workable plan. Clearly, in a 15-minute interaction, the physician cannot glean information in all of the relevant domains identified by the authors. Rather, the authors focus on the physician's ability to identify "red flags," which suggest the need for further probing to understand the context of the patient's life. The "red flags" may be in the form of statements made by the patients or communicated through the patient's behavior, for example, frequently missing appointments. With physician and institutional review board approval, they audiotaped the interactions between "standardized patients" (actors playing patients) and real patients with physicians. In analyzing the tapes, they developed a coding system to identify the outcomes of each encounter, called "4C"— Content Coding for Contextualization of Care. Their coding asks the following questions: Does the patient demonstrate a possible contextual factor which may be a red flag? If there is a red flag, does the physician ask about it? If the patient revealed a contextual factor, was it in response to a probe by the physician? If there is a contextual factor, did the physician address it in the care plan?

Unlike most areas in the quality of care, the patient chart is not a reliable source for identifying failures to deal with patient context. The authors provide thoughtful and interesting approaches to the use of audiotapes to record physician–patient interactions using standardized patients in experimental models and actual patients in quality improvement efforts. The studies indicate that a significant portion of care plans are flawed because they do not adequately address patient context, even when "red flags" are raised by the patient's comments or behavior. Controlled studies of learning by medical students indicated that they can learn how to identify aspects of patient context and take these into consideration in caring for the patient. Aggressive efforts to educate residents and practitioners showed that their awareness of patient context can be improved and health plans modified to reflect this context. However, it is as yet unclear what the longevity of the learned behaviors may be.

Audio studies are complex operationally, technically, and ethically. As the authors point out, in many other industries, recordings are made in order to assess quality; but this technique is a relatively new and infrequently applied strategy in medicine. Their recordings yielded information about a broad spectrum of physician communication skills and strategies which, at times, were appalling. Frequent interruption of the patient, failure to hear what the patient is saying, use of a rote checklist to obtain a history, and a complete failure to understand why the patient has come to see the physician and how the patient perceives their problem are only a few of the weaknesses which these studies revealed.

Although some of these studies were conducted in the offices of private practice physicians, many were conducted within Department of Veterans Affairs (VA) hospitals. The special issues confronted by VA patients and the structure of the provider workforce in the VA raise questions about the generalizability of the research findings in this population. However, the work is extremely useful in identifying methodologies, with appropriate modifications, which may be important in improving education and performance during a wide variety of patient–doctor interactions.

To what extent is the concept of contextualizing care in and of itself an important notion? Currently, there is widespread commitment to the concept of patient-centered care (i.e., care that is respectful and responsive to individual patient preferences, needs, and values). Don Berwick has defined patient-centered care as "The experience (to the extent the informed, individual patient desires it) of transparency, individualization, recognition, respect, dignity and choice in all matters without exception, related to one's personal circumstances in relationships in healthcare."[2] This definition emphasizes the importance of contextualizing care as described by Weiner and Schwartz.

If completely implemented, patient-centered care would include all of the considerations of contextual care. However, the concept of patient-centered care is so broad that methods to evaluate it require attention to specific aspects. Contextualizing care provides just such an opportunity and allows application across the broad range of domains identified by the authors. At the same time, it has offered opportunities to develop methodologies that could be applied much more widely. The detailed description of how the authors undertook their investigations and dealt with the ethical and bureaucratic issues associated with audiotaping of patient–doctor exchanges is an important contribution to understanding how to improve care in a manner that does not ordinarily present itself in the medical records.

Another important contribution from these studies is the understanding that addressing some aspects of patient-centered care need not dramatically increase the amount of time required by the patient–doctor interaction. The studies also highlight the challenges associated with bringing other health professionals into the process of patient-centered care.

Hopefully, as these methodologies are refined, they can be applied more broadly in other parts of the health care–delivery system, both as parts of investigations and as continuous quality improvement. Medical educators have been writing and working extensively about methods to improve communication skills for students at every level of their career. The results of the studies reported in this book indicate that much needs to be done if the patient–doctor interaction can live up to its expectations across the health-care system. The methods proposed by the authors offer some real opportunities to accomplish this goal. Their explicit identification of the context of the patient's situation is a central part of the patient–physician interaction. The subsequent plan for the patient and physician arising from the context is an important contribution. The authors' experience with audiotaping and analyzing the recorded interactions opens important new avenues to improve the quality of health care.

Kenneth Shine, MD
Past President, Institute of Medicine of the National Academies

NOTES

1. Kohn LT, Corrigan J, Donaldson MS. To err is human: building a safer health system. Washington, DC: National Academies Press; 2000.
2. Berwick, D. What patient-centered should mean: confessions of an extremist. Health Aff. 2009;28(4):w555–w565. Retrieved March 25, 2011. https://www.health affairs.org/doi/10.1377/hlthaff.28.4.w555.

Introduction: Some Context

Our fascination with the topic of contextualizing care took root at the turn of the millennium when the evidence-based medicine movement had emerged. We noticed that although medical residents were skilled at identifying the latest studies and guidelines, their care plans often didn't seem appropriate once one considered the life challenges some of their patients were facing. We'd see, for instance, a patient with poorly controlled diabetes put on a higher dose of a medication they weren't taking (Insulin Glargine), rather than a less costly alternative (e.g., NPH), when the context was that they couldn't afford it. We coined the term "contextual error" to describe these kinds of mistakes.

We suspected that contextual errors could have significant implications for patient care and that they were not captured using existing methods for identifying other types of medical error. We had so many questions: How common are they? What impact do they have, particularly on health-care outcomes and costs? Are they preventable and, if so, how? And, perhaps most importantly for anyone seeking answers, how are they detected and their effects measured? This book is about what we've learned through studies pursuing these and related questions. Whereas in the first edition we described at length the challenges of conducting research that requires novel methods of direct, often covert, observation of care, in this edition we focus more on the practical application of research findings for improving this unmeasured and underappreciated dimension of quality of care. We've also conducted several new studies and explain their implications.

Because much of what we describe is new to many readers, we begin here with a tour through the overarching concepts and methods that are explored in further depth in the chapters that follow. It's useful to start by considering some of the long-standing terms and descriptors that have emerged over the years to describe attention to the non-biomedical aspects of medicine including "the art of medicine," biopsychosocial medicine, the "judicious and reasonable use" of current best evidence, patient-centered medicine, social care, narrative medicine, cultural competence, and social determinants of health (SDOH). Of course, each refers to something somewhat different. What they share, however, is the idea that medical need and medical care occur within the broader context of patients' lives. That may seem self-evident, but in the 1970s when George Engel described the biopsychosocial model, in which he introduced general systems theory as a framework for broadening the biomedical perspective to include social, psychological, and behavioral dimensions, he observed that much of the profession was "unreceptive if not hostile" to deviations from the biomedical model. Engel quoted an authority who reflected the thinking of the times, calling for "a disentanglement of the organic elements of disease from the psychosocial elements of human malfunction" and that "medicine should deal with the former only."[1]

Academic medicine has begun to advance beyond that perspective. In 2019 the National Academies of Sciences, Engineering, and Medicine released a report titled *Integrating Social Care into the Delivery of Health Care*,[2] and medical schools now incorporate social medicine topics in their curricula. Still, little is known about how these concepts are applied, at a practical level, when the exam room door is closed and physician and patient are alone together. If you were a fly on the wall, observing a medical encounter, what would you need to see to say that "social care was/was not just practiced" or the use of research evidence was/was not "judicious," or "that doctor took/missed an opportunity to address SDOH"? And even if you reached a conclusion, would others share it? And, finally, if they did, would these assessments predict patients' outcomes? To answer these questions, you'd have to agree on what to look for, how it represents what you are trying to measure, and how you'd know it when you saw it.

To our knowledge, these questions have not been previously addressed. George Engel did not attempt to operationalize "biopsychosocial medicine" as a performance measure. Rather, "biopsychosocial" is a conceptual framework for talking about health and health care beyond the biomedical, not for systematically evaluating individual medical encounters. In fact, the very notion of a performance measure for "biopsychosocial care" may seem paradoxical. It's one thing to ascertain whether a clinician applies biomedical knowledge appropriately and another whether they appropriately adapt care to each patient's particular life situation. For instance, it's relatively straightforward to evaluate primary care physicians based on their implementation of evidence-based diabetes screening guidelines for high-risk patients. In contrast, how does one evaluate the response of a physician to a particular patient with diabetes who can no longer manage their condition because they lost their job and health insurance?

In formulating an answer, we find it helpful to contrast two scenarios: First, imagine a physician who identifies the underlying financial problem and switches the patient to lower-cost medications such as generics. Because the care plan addressed the non-biomedical *context* for the patient's deteriorating clinical state, we say they "contextualized care." Now imagine the physician, instead, misses the signs that their patient is struggling with costs and, unhelpfully, prescribes additional medications, further driving up costs. Because the clinician's error is due to an inattention to the context, we call it a "contextual error." Conceptually, comparing these two approaches illustrates why it is feasible to distinguish between care that attends to patient context and care that does not.

And yet such variation in practice, despite its implications, is not captured by any of the existing required or recommended health-care quality measures. The most widely used tools, the Healthcare Effectiveness Data and Information Set (HEDIS˚) measures, rely on data extracted from surveys, medical charts, and insurance claims. It is not possible from such sources to assess whether clinicians are identifying and addressing the challenges that individual patients face that complicate their care.

Things that are not measured are usually not a priority. Perhaps not surprisingly, medical training—especially the residency years immediately following medical school—heavily emphasizes efficient task completion rather than figuring out what's really best for the individual patient. These tasks can be distilled to assessing a patient's clinical status and ordering labs, consults, radiological studies, screening tests, and medication refills—and then completing a note that meets billing requirements and justifies whatever interventions occurred. Attending physicians nod approvingly when residents seem both efficient and evidence-based. And yet, how often would such care no longer seem sufficient if you had pertinent information about the patient's life situation?

Without a meaningful and scalable method of assessing contextualization of care, calls for the judicious application of research evidence, improved patient-centered care, or attention to SDOH will have limited effect. Our early work focused on tackling that problem.

BECOMING THE FLY ON THE WALL

To assess physician attention (or lack of attention) to non-biomedical aspects of patient care, we needed a way to hear their conversations with their patients—ideally when they are behaving naturally, unaware that they are being observed. We adopted two methods: an experimental one in which actors portray patients incognito (the "unannounced standardized patient" [USP] method) and an observational one in which real patients volunteer to covertly audio-record their visits. We have extensively employed both, after gaining the trust of participating clinicians and patients. We adhere to detailed ethical and legal requirements.

Listening in on a medical encounter feels like a rare privilege—and it is. Of the myriad studies of health care taking place at any given time, most are based on secondary sources such as medical claims data, data extracted from the electronic health record (EHR), and survey data. Too few have employed direct observation of the clinician in practice. Although we have engaged over 6,000 real patients to record their visits in several health-care settings and have published our findings frequently, we have come upon few other published reports based on direct covert observation of real medical encounters. This is a concerning gap because much of the interaction during a medical encounter—the beneficial and the potentially harmful—is never documented in the EHR. Hence, a great deal of variation in quality is currently unmeasured and, as a result, cannot be characterized and addressed.

How is it that so few study and assess health-care delivery by observing it? Many believe the hurdles are overwhelming or that the payoff for the effort is too low. Some seem incredulous when they hear that we have engaged thousands of patients to covertly record their medical visits with the knowledge and support of their doctors. Indeed, the challenges are formidable both because of the anxiety that direct covert observation can generate and because the logistics are complex.

Overcoming those hurdles opened a window into the exam room. Almost at once, we noticed discrepancies between what we were hearing on recordings and what was documented in the medical record. When health professionals enter data into the EHR, they are constrained by time, billing requirements, and their own recall and biases. As a result, there is a gap—perhaps a chasm—between health care as documented and health care as actually delivered. On audio recordings, we've heard countless instances of patients sharing information about personal circumstances vital to care planning (e.g., the loss of a caregiver or new competing responsibilities) that are overlooked or disregarded. The medical records for these visits, however, reveal few of these lapses (e.g., the physician notes only that a condition is poorly controlled). Conversely, we also hear clinicians who astutely identify and address relevant context without documenting what they learned or did.

ANALYZING WHAT YOU OBSERVE

Recording visits is only a first step. Unlike the organized taxonomy of diagnostic and procedural codes, a conversation is a morass of unfiltered information. Physician–patient communication is commonly analyzed using one of two strategies: inductive approaches such as grounded theory—in which researchers listen for themes that emerge, from which they can draw inferences—or interaction analysis. Interaction analysis systematically codes the *process* of communication. Process measures tabulate turn-taking, interruptions, pauses, backchanneling ("Uh-huh, right"), socioemotional utterances, and so on.[3] After exploring both, we concluded that neither strategy is suited to assessing contextualization of care. We sought to answer questions such as "Did the physician pursue specific clues that their patient is struggling with a life challenge?" and "Did they attempt to incorporate what they learned into their care plan?" Specifically, our interest is in the *logic* of a conversation between physician and patient rather than the process. To follow that logical thread, and in a manner that could be reliably reproduced by different listeners, we had to develop a new coding system, focused on the content rather than the process of communication.

Importantly, we weren't looking at all the content—only that which is essential to care planning. After all, clinicians often have only a few minutes with patients. But where to draw the line? What does a physician need to elicit from a patient to provide contextualized care? To appreciate the coding challenge, consider the physician caring for the patient briefly introduced above who lost control of their diabetes when they became unemployed. Initially, all the physician sees is an increased glycated hemoglobin level, noted at the start of the visit. Effective care requires figuring out that the patient's setback occurred after they lost health insurance coverage for their costly prescription medications. But the more one asks, the more one learns, like peeling back the layers of an onion: It turned out that the loss occurred when their and their partner's small trucking business had recently failed. And the trucking business failed because they had to lease vehicles instead of purchasing them, resulting in higher fixed costs. They had been unable to purchase the trucks because they could not secure loans despite solid credit, a common problem for Black-owned businesses. Hence, the larger context for poorly controlled blood sugar here includes the health insurance system and the effects of systemic racism on a patient who happened to be Black.

Although understanding the larger context helps the physician appreciate their patient's situation, not all of the information is essential to planning their care. For instance, it is essential for the physician to know that the patient's loss of diabetes control coincides with loss of health insurance and that there are less costly alternatives to the medication they are currently taking. It is not necessary for the physician to know, however, about the failure of the trucking business and its root causes. Although this larger picture provides insight and perspective that could inform policy changes, it is outside what one might call the physician's basic irreducible minimum for treating this patient. It isn't necessary to know why their business failed to realize they need affordable medication.

Our body of work revolves around the concept of "patient life context," or "patient context" for short. Patient context is defined as "everything that is expressed outside of a patient's skin that is relevant to planning their care." An alternate definition that is less abstract but also less precise is "Patient or caregiver circumstances and behaviors that are relevant to planning care." Note that both conclude with the phrase "relevant to planning care."

Contextualizing care is a four-step cognitive process. Step 1 involves recognizing clues of patient context, termed "contextual red flags." Loss of control of diabetes, for instance, is a contextual red flag because it should prompt the clinician to wonder whether something has changed in a patient's life that has disrupted their ability to take their medication as directed or eat an appropriate diet. Step 2 is asking patients about contextual red flags, as in "Ms. Davis, I notice that your diabetes no longer seems to be well managed. Can you tell me what's changed?" We call these inquiries about contextual red flags "contextual probing." Step 3 is listening to the patient's response and identifying a specific contextual factor if present (i.e., the patient context). For Ms. Davis, this was loss of health insurance. And finally, step 4 is taking the contextual factor into account when planning the patient's care. That is the end goal: to "contextualize care." For instance, ordering less costly alternatives to the medications Ms. Davis is taking to manage her diabetes represents a contextualized care plan. In sum, the schema is as follows:

Contextual red flag → Contextual probe → Contextual factor →
Contextualized care plan

Tracking each step enables a trained audio coder to ascertain whether a clinician contextualizes a care plan. The coder first identifies any contextual red flags and then observes whether the clinician completed the remaining three steps for each of them. Alternatively, patients sometimes tell their physician about a contextual factor without any prompting (i.e., no contextual probe). For instance, Ms. Davis might comment during the visit that "it's been tough affording my medication since I lost my health insurance coverage." In such instances, the coding process is even more straightforward:

Contextual factor → Contextualized care plan

Tracking these steps also enables coders to identify and document contextual errors when they occur. A contextual error occurs whenever a contextual factor is identified (either as a response to a contextual probe or when volunteered by the patient) but not addressed in the care plan. For instance, if the clinician heard Ms. Davis say that she had lost her health insurance, either with or without being asked, and nevertheless responded by adding more medication that the patient already couldn't afford, the coder would document a contextual error.

This rather simple framework enabled us to develop a system for analyzing audio-recorded encounters, called "Content Coding for Contextualization of Care," or "4C" for short. 4C provides the tool that was needed: Non-clinician coders with a few days of training can efficiently and reliably identify contextual red flags, probes, and factors and, finally, recognize whether care plans are contextualized. Coders can also identify if a contextual error has occurred.

One of the rules 4C coders are taught is to count any care plan that attempts to address a contextual factor as contextualized, even if they think the clinician could have come up with something better. For instance, 4C will give credit for any attempt to get Ms. Davis on a treatment plan she can afford, even if it appears less likely to work than other options. This practice simplifies coding, enabling high inter-rater agreement, essential to any performance measure. In addition, it builds credibility. Few accuse us of being nit-picky. This is especially helpful when we code a contextual error. For instance, few would argue that sending Ms. Davis home with medications she can't afford is effective care. Because a goal of our work is to convince clinicians to change how they practice, the data need to be convincing to them as well as to our research colleagues.

The following chapter outline provides an overview of where the concepts introduced above appear in greater detail and how they fit together. We hope readers find this small amount of redundancy helpful rather than tiresome. While preparing this edition, we produced a series of videos, available on YouTube, called the Fireside Chat Series on Contextualization of Care, in which we discuss key concepts and skills and illustrate them with examples. A link to the playlist is in the references.[4] Throughout the book we reference specific videos as applicable.

CHAPTER OUTLINE

The first four chapters, under the heading Part I, "The Problem," describe what we know about physician attention to patient life context, how we know it, and why it matters. Chapter 1, titled "Observing the Problem," is structured around a series of case examples that illustrate what happens when clinicians overlook patient context and how care planning changes when they finally take it into account. We also propose some hypotheses about why failures to incorporate patient context into care planning occur. We consider how providing patient care entails knowing what questions to ask patients and how to ask them. We conclude with an illustration of why contextualizing care is not a linear "checklist" process. At its best, it emerges out of an engaged interaction between two individuals working together to solve problems, one in the healing role and the other seeking better health through health care. "Engagement" is an important concept that describes a particular kind of interaction between individuals, and we devote some time to it later in the book.

Chapter 2, "Measuring the Problem," transitions from anecdotes and hypotheses to systematic inquiry, describing our early research. We classify contextual error as a subtype of medical error that has been overlooked because it is not detectable utilizing conventional methods for detecting error. We describe the conundrum we found ourselves in, trying to track something that usually leaves no footprint. After considering several options, we decided to observe physician decision-making directly by sending unannounced standardized "secret shopper" patients (USPs) undercover into doctors' practices to portray cases that challenge physicians to think contextually. Doing so, however, posed a considerable challenge, including manipulating the medical record to create fake patient medical charts, training actors to adopt the personae of real patients while adhering to a script, and gaining the trust of physicians who consented not to know when a fake patient is covertly recording them. We also needed the support of several senior leaders in the Veterans Health Administration system—where we collected much of our data—who took steps to protect us from larger forces that wanted to shut this groundbreaking project down. What we learned from this work is that even when patients drop hints that there are life factors interfering with their care, doctors often miss them, instead sending them out with plans that look appropriate on paper but, in fact, are not if one takes into account the context.

Having documented that physicians overlook relevant context more often than not in an experimental model, our next step was to see how often context matters in actual practice. To do that, we had to transition from employing actors with contrived problems, each customized to test clinician attention to context, to recruiting real patients with real problems and asking them to carry hidden audio recorders. Chapter 3 describes this phase of our work. What we stood to gain was insight about how often effective care really hinges on a personalized approach in which individual life circumstances are a key factor in planning. We also were interested in whether the poor performance we observed when clinicians interacted with actors was, in fact, representative of care real patients receive in practice. Our title for Chapter 3, "The Problem Is Everywhere," hints at what we found.

Going from fake to real patients changed what we could measure: With USPs we could assess and compare physician performance under conditions we determined. With real patients, in contrast, there was no way to know what patient context, if any, would come up during a visit—what vital information regarding life situations and potential obstacles to effective care would emerge. Hence, we had to develop a flexible and reliable system for assessing the clinician's attention to contextual information when we would not know the context in advance. With the introduction of real patients, however, we now had an opportunity to compare the health-care outcomes of patients whose care clinicians contextualized compared with those whose care plans were inattentive to their life needs and circumstances.

As with our strategy of introducing fake patients into the clinical setting, enlisting real patients to carry concealed audio recorders into their visits posed a set of challenges we had to address. Whereas others have employed USPs in the clinical setting, as far as we are aware asking real patients to covertly record their encounters was a first. We discuss how we addressed the ethical and legal issues as well as the potential concerns of participants, clinicians, and patients alike.

Chapter 4, "What We Hear That Physicians Don't," is a bit of a technical dive into how our research team works with the data collected from audio-recorded encounters. In particular, elaborating on the overview provided above, we describe the coding system we developed, 4C. By coding content, in contrast to coding of process, 4C requires following the thread and logic of a conversation. In this chapter we also discuss why we had to develop 4C, namely, because other approaches to assessing communication that are commonly employed in doctor–patient communication research do not capture information on whether clinicians are actually paying attention to and addressing key information that comes up during the encounter.

Part II, titled "Solutions," comprising the remaining chapters, takes stock of what we have learned about the challenges of contextualizing care and how we can use that knowledge both to reduce contextual errors and to empower patients to ensure that they receive care that is not only based on clinical evidence but adapted to their needs and circumstances. We begin with "High versus Low Performers," in which we ask, essentially, "What makes a clinician good at this?" Although our studies were not designed to answer the "Why?" question, after analyzing thousands of encounters, we have identified six attributes that lead a physician either to overlook context or to recognize and incorporate it; and Chapter 5 is where we share them.

Chapter 6, "Better Teaching, Better Doctors," describes an educational program we developed and assessed, using a research method most associated with the study of clinical interventions—the randomized controlled trial. We tested whether a brief experiential curriculum could prepare physicians to be more effective at contextualizing care, as measured by actors role-playing standardized patients in a performance laboratory. We worked with fourth-year medical school students for this project because they seemed at the right point in the developmental trajectory of a physician—not too junior to appreciate the complexities of patient care but not so far along as to be irrevocably fixed in their ways. Although the results of this study were gratifying—we saw improvement—later work with more rigorous measures revealed important limitations. In a subsequent study we describe, residents were evaluated with both standardized patients in the lab and

USPs in the actual practice setting. The results in the lab were like those of medical students, but the results in practice were markedly different. We explore this "skills-to-performance" gap and its implications.

One of the lessons of Chapter 6 is that teaching the skills to contextualize care is not enough to change how physicians practice. Changing practice requires ongoing feedback and/or the use of technology at the point of care. In Chapter 7, "Is Lasting Change Possible?," we describe three different interventions we've developed and tested. The first entailed sharing with physicians and other health-care professionals ongoing data on their performance at contextualizing care, based on analysis of audio recordings of encounters with their patients. In the second we employed USPs in a plan–do–study–act cycle. These interventions are like "holding a mirror up" to the clinician so that they can see what their care looks like, both the good (contextualized care) and the bad (contextual errors), and adapt accordingly. In the third intervention we designed clinical decision support tools in the EHR that guide physicians to contextualize care, drawing on data provided by patients before the visits and from their medical record.

Chapter 8, "What We Can't Measure That Matters," is about variations in how clinicians attend to context that we don't know how to measure. In particular, 4C does not assess how physicians employ themselves as an intervention when patients have certain emotions or behaviors that complicate their care. One of us has recently written a book, *On Becoming a Healer: The Journey from Patient Care to Caring about Your Patients*, that explores, in part, the difficult-to-measure elements of an optimal clinical interaction.[5] We are indebted to our late colleague Simon Auster for his insights on the themes discussed, especially the description of open and full engagement with boundary clarity as the ideal approach to clinical interactions that attend to patient context.

In Chapter 9, "Bringing Context Back into Care," we argue that in an era in which home visits and deep continuity across generations between a doctor and their patients is uncommon, contextualization of care must be taught, reinforced, and measured to change practice. And for that to happen, methods of direct observation of care must be widely adopted.

Throughout this work we describe case interactions to illustrate various points. We've removed identifiers and, in some cases, altered facts to protect the identities of patients. If you choose to read this book from cover to cover, we hope you will experience some of the surprise and discovery we have experienced. One of the practical challenges we faced in writing this book as two authors is narrative voice. For nearly two decades we have collaborated closely on this work, bringing different skills and fulfilling complementary roles. Perhaps the most natural way of telling the story would have been to imagine that the two of us were sitting around an open fire with you, the reader. Each of us would take turns, referring to the other by name when relating anecdotes. We might alternate from Alan telling how "Saul went out to meet with a group of physicians in a small suburb to see if we could send them fake patients" to Saul explaining that "Alan suggested we e-mail physicians to see whether they could tell us which of their patients was fake." Although this style works well around a campfire, our editor convinced us that it is not a good way to talk to an audience from the pages of a book. Hence, throughout, we have adopted the third-person plural, "we." In fact, it is often just one of us to whom we are referring. If it sounds like something a doctor would do, it is probably Saul. If it sounds like something a research methodologist would do, it is probably Alan. If it sounds like something that neither could do alone, it probably was both.

Finally, a comment about names and identifiers. We have changed the names of nearly all clinicians and staff, retaining only those whose identities and titles were significant to the narrative and who agreed to be named. In all patient descriptions we have altered not only names but identifiers in order to assure privacy.

NOTES

1. Engel GL. The need for a new medical model: a challenge for biomedicine. Science. 1977;196(4286):129–136.
2. National Academies of Sciences, Engineering, and Medicine 2019. Integrating social care into the delivery of health care: moving upstream to improve the nation's health. Washington, DC: National Academies Press. https://doi.org/10.17226/25467.
3. Roter D, Larson S. The Roter interaction analysis system (RIAS): utility and flexibility for analysis of medical interactions. Patient Educ Couns. 2002;46(4):243–251. DOI: 10.1016/s0738-3991(02)00012-5.
4. Weiner SJ. Contextualizing care: fireside chat series. YouTube, February 6, 2022. https://youtube.com/playlist?list=PL9-b6XZZMupzmVuuwn1Ipph0dpI1fxx2d. Accessed May 25, 2022.
5. Weiner SJ. On becoming a healer: the journey from patient care to caring about your patients. Johns Hopkins University Press; 2020.

PART I

The Problem

Observing the Problem

By a mere technician I mean a man who understands everything about his job except its ultimate purpose.

—Sir Richard W. Livingstone (attrib.)[1]

INTRODUCING CONTEXT: WHAT IS MISSING FROM BIOMEDICALLY FOCUSED CARE?

The term "biomedical" is defined as "involving biological, medical, and physical science."[2] What is excluded from a biomedical focus is the surrounding context, that is, "the situation within which something exists or happens, and that can help explain it."[3] This includes the life circumstances that contribute to a particular patient's clinical presentation. Without attention to context, clinical care has a narrow technical focus, which can lead to a failure to achieve its ultimate purpose.

Consider, for instance, Amelia Garcia, a Spanish-speaking 62-year-old woman with kidney failure who returned to the University of Illinois (UI Health) Medical Center emergency department (ED) repeatedly because she'd missed her hemodialysis. Each time she showed up in the emergency room, doctors would select a therapy based on the results of her blood tests and electrocardiogram (ECG). They focused on what was going on inside her body, including her elevated potassium (hyperkalemia) and changes to electrical conduction in her heart. At her fourth visit, when her serum potassium was nearly 7.0 mmol/L, a life-threatening level, her ECG showed peaked t-waves and, more ominously, early widening of the QRS complex, a precursor of a potentially lethal arrhythmia. As on prior occasions, the ED staff inserted an IV into her arm. To manage the hyperkalemia, she was treated initially with calcium gluconate, which immediately stabilizes the heart muscle to reduce the chance of a fatal rhythm disturbance, followed by other medications which help drive serum potassium levels down temporarily. She was then transferred to the nephrology unit for hemodialysis. As in the past, the plan was to send her home later that day or the following morning, her emergency managed, with reminders not to miss dialysis again and a warning that doing so could be fatal. ED staff sometimes refer to patients like Ms. Garcia who turn up repeatedly as "frequent flyers." In her medical record, she was described as "hemodialysis noncompliant" at each previous visit.

But this visit was different. Before she was discharged, a medical student caring for her asked her why she missed her dialysis. Through another student who was bilingual, Ms. Garcia explained that she lived with her daughter who worked two jobs to support them, and a 10-year-old grandson with an unrelated renal condition who had had a kidney transplant. She took him regularly to see a pediatric nephrologist, also at UI Health.

Ms. Garcia explained that she is dialyzed at a site that is not only far from her home but also far from UI Health. The Medicaid-funded transportation service that she relies on will pick her up at her home and take her to and from dialysis, but there is no way for her to get directly from the dialysis center to the medical center when her grandson needs care. Hence, she is often forced to choose between her grandson's medical needs and her own—and she prioritizes his.

When the inpatient team raised with her the possibility of moving her hemodialysis over to their own on-site outpatient dialysis unit, Ms. Garcia responded enthusiastically. She had not been aware she could get long-term dialysis at the medical center. She commented that she could then bring her son to his nephrology appointment on the same days she came for hemodialysis. That would solve her transportation problem and enable her to get the prescribed three times weekly hemodialysis. The medical team contacted the social worker who managed hemodialysis, and she facilitated the transfer of care. A review of Ms. Garcia's medical record almost a year later showed no subsequent ED visits or hospital admissions.

INATTENTION TO CONTEXT: DOCTORS WITH BLINDERS

Reflecting on how the physicians cared for Ms. Garcia, two major opposing themes emerge: On the one hand, they were responsive to the biomedical aspects of her care. They knew that bad things happen inside the body when patients miss their hemodialysis and held themselves accountable for evaluating her clinically each time she arrived in the ED. This process involved asking relevant questions such as, "What metabolic abnormalities should I consider in this patient?" They sought and found the answers, then intervened promptly to correct those that were life-threatening.

On the other hand, they exhibited a distinct lack of curiosity about *why* someone who evidenced no other self-destructive behaviors would repeatedly return to the unappealing environment of a crowded urban emergency room with a self-inflicted life-threatening condition. They repeatedly failed to ask, "Ms. Garcia, can you tell us why you keep missing your hemodialysis?" Instead, they assigned a generic label to her behavior—"non-compliant"—and applied a generic response: to admonish her to do better next time. Although they got the technical, or biomedical, aspects of her care right each time she came to the hospital, it took several admissions before they considered the surrounding context, eliciting the essential information necessary to prevent the recurrent "relapses" that required emergency interventions.

Sending Ms. Garcia home without identifying and addressing the life circumstance that accounted for her missing dialysis constituted a kind of medical error called a "contextual error." A contextual error occurs when a care plan is biomedically sound but nevertheless inappropriate because of a failure to take into account relevant patient context. Not seeing patient context is akin to wearing blinders, the small screens attached to a horse's bridle to prevent them from getting distracted by what's around them. Horses, however, have riders who can see and react to what's around them. When physicians have blinders on, there is no one with a wide-angle view perched above them to redirect their actions.

The blinders physicians wear are not, of course, physical. Rather, they are imposed by a set of expectations physicians internalize during their training about what information about patients matters. Understanding what is going on inside the patient—literally—matters. Understanding their behavior is deprioritized. When patients are not "doing what they were told" they are regarded, simply, as "non-compliant." The possibility that there is a backstory is lost.

To further appreciate how contextual errors occur, let's return to the patient who had stopped taking her diabetes medication because of cost (described in the introduction). In addition, Ms. Davis—as we'll call her—had declined what her physicians had told her was necessary surgery—a coronary artery bypass graft surgery, after she'd suffered a myocardial infarction and was diagnosed with triple-vessel heart disease. A cardiologist documented that she had "refused" recommended care and indicated no plans to proceed at this time. The context, however, revealed a more complex picture: As discussed, Ms. Davis and her husband, Ray Davis, had recently lost their family business, in which they leased and drove trucks. Probably because they were Black, they'd been unable to acquire the credit to purchase their vehicles; without the banking relationships, they had been unsuccessful at obtaining funds through the COVID-19 Paycheck Protection Program. Paying leasing fees resulted in considerable financial and personal stress, risk of foreclosure on their home, and even food insecurity. With the loss of the business came loss of health insurance. Ms. Davis applied for Medicaid, which pays retroactively, but was still wary of racking up further debt. In addition to loss of the business, her husband had suffered a stroke 6 months earlier while recovering from COVID-19. She now assisted him with many of his activities of daily living, including transferring from bed to chair and bathing.

Ms. Davis had stopped renewing some of her medications because of the cost. She missed appointments when she couldn't find anyone to look after her husband. Her reasons for declining surgery, however, dated back further. About 5 years earlier, when her husband was recovering from back surgery after an accident, she'd seen him suffer because his physicians did not adequately treat his pain. He'd been reluctant to complain, fearing they'd label him as drug-seeking. She did not want to go through what he had with her own surgery. Rather, she'd adopted a fatalistic attitude, praying and saying, "I'm in God's hands."

The failure of Ms. Davis' physicians to identify and address the relevant context in her life was a contextual error. The consequence was a missed opportunity to address barriers to medical and appointment adherence and needed surgery. How might her physicians have cared for her differently if they identified and addressed the context? Would they have referred her to social work to arrange respite care for her husband—especially when she had medical appointments? In addition to switching her to lower cost insulin, might they have connected her with the hospital financial services office to assist her in getting onto Medicaid and to show her that the pharmacy would bill Medicaid directly? Might they have reviewed with her their plan for managing post-operative pain, acknowledging how racist views about pain tolerance have often led to undertreatment of pain in Black patients?

Given the relevance of the information to planning appropriate care, how might the physicians caring for her have efficiently acquired the context needed to provide her with appropriate care, a process we term "contextualizing care"? What clues would they have needed to recognize, and what questions would they have had to ask? And, finally, why didn't they seek to better understand her situation? Quite literally: What were they thinking?

STUDYING PHYSICIAN DECISION-MAKING: THE IMPORTANCE OF EXAMINING THE MUNDANE

Accounts of great physicians, including television portrayals, typically focus on diagnostic acumen or surgical skill. TV drama doctors exhibit expert knowledge and skill, are highly methodical, and uncover rare diseases. In real life, however, most medical encounters do not involve making rare diagnoses because such conditions are rare (by definition); furthermore, diagnosing a rare condition is no longer quite so hard because medical technology has made the inner workings of the body ever more transparent. The more pervasive challenge in medical practice is managing common and often chronic conditions well. It's not typically answering questions like, "Does this patient have porphyria cutanea tarda?" but "What can I do to help Ms. Davis get her diabetes under control despite her difficulty paying for medications and the stresses of caring for her disabled partner?" Just to frame such a question requires recognizing the clinical relevance of the quotidian life of the patient. When a patient comments, for instance, "Boy, it's been tough since I lost my job," does the doctor appreciate that it is a clue about why the patient has lost control of their blood pressure? Does the doctor ask, "How has it been difficult since you lost your job?" and discover that the patient can no longer afford the brand-name antihypertensive cardioselective beta blocker they were prescribed? Does the doctor use this information to prescribe a cheaper generic?

In contrast to rare conditions like porphyria cutanea tarda, conditions such as financial hardship, competing responsibilities, and a loss of trust in the health-care system are common. Although relatively mundane from the vantage point of a professional who has spent over a decade acquiring specialized knowledge, such information is essential to planning effective care. Hence, effective doctors care about patient context.[4]

Despite its centrality to effective medical practice, the capacity to identify and address patient context—to contextualize care—is not measured. This double standard in which physicians are expected to rigorously examine biomedical aspects of care but can disregard patient context is reflected in how physicians are evaluated and trained. Students are encouraged to get to know their patients and to feel empathy for their situations, but that is not the same as teaching a systematic process for identifying and incorporating relevant patient context into clinical care. This gap in training, in turn, shapes (as it reflects) the profession's understanding of its role—with unfortunate consequences. In our work as educators of medical students and residents, we have seen repeatedly how physicians' views of their roles and responsibilities, when limited to a narrow technical focus that is inattentive to context, can undermine care.

FAULTING THE PATIENT: THE FUNDAMENTAL ATTRIBUTION ERROR

Inattention to context represents a lack of curiosity. It may, in part, be due to what psychologists refer to as the "fundamental attribution error" (FAE), which is, essentially, a failure to consider the complex situational reasons other people apparently behave irrationally or inappropriately and instead attribute their behavior to a fundamental flaw in their character.[5] This is likely the reason why the health-care team responsible for Ms. Garcia did not think to ask, "Why in the world is this woman, who seems reasonably intelligent, coming to an unpleasant place—our ED—so often for a problem that is easy to avoid?" Notably, the FAE is not one that we often make when thinking about ourselves because we can readily see—and we experience—the context that shapes our own behavior. Ms. Garcia had no difficulty explaining why she was missing her hemodialysis. She only needed to be asked. Perhaps because she was unaware that there were things the health-care team could do to help her, and perhaps because of the language barrier, she never volunteered the information.

When the FAE leads doctors to attribute patient behaviors to a patient's personality rather than to their life circumstances, it can lead them to judge and label patients. A resident physician described his patient, Melanie Richards, as "anti-social" to his supervising attending, noting that she did not even acknowledge him when he came into the exam room. When the attending subsequently entered, he extended his hand in greeting to Ms. Richards, who was perched on an exam table; and, sure enough, she did not reciprocate. Initially, the attending did not say anything and proceeded with the interaction, noticing along the way that she seemed pleasant. Near the end of the visit, he asked her why she had not taken his hand when he had entered and offered it to her. Initially, she looked puzzled. It turned out that she had lost her peripheral vision several years earlier from a pituitary tumor that had been removed, and the door through which the doctors entered and approached her was outside her field of vision. The resident's assessment that the patient was unfriendly reflected an ingrained association between a social convention (the handshake) and an individual's personal qualities. The resident did not question the discrepancy between the patient's apparently rude behavior and her otherwise genial demeanor. Had the discrepancy not been explored with a simple question, her doctors would have regarded her as disengaged, a perception that could have shaped how they related to her, potentially undermining her care.

The tendency to judge a patient rather than explore the context for their behavior leads to false conclusions—including that they are not responsible (Garcia) or rude (Richards) or, in the following example, "demanding": A patient suffering from chronic back pain said, "Doctor, I've got to have some oxycodone for my pain" because they had heard that this particular (often abused) medication works for pain. The doctor interpreted the request as "demanding" or "drug-seeking" when it was really just a call for help—and that call went unanswered as the physician lectured the patient on why narcotics are not appropriate for treating chronic pain but neglected to explore the patient's job responsibilities lifting heavy equipment. What the physician failed to appreciate, because they did not try to understand how the patient came to make this request, is that patients simply have needs, such as treatment for pain, and that they often express those needs by proposing treatments that they've heard are effective. This patient wasn't seeking drugs. He was seeking relief.

Judging patients rather than exploring context can become a way of viewing others. The rationalization that patients are "just demanding," for instance, can extend to situations where the drug sought is not even pleasant. Consider Mr. Eli Gates, an African American Vietnam veteran in his sixties, who came in with his wife requesting antibiotics for what he believed was an infected tooth. He was seen initially by Dr. Jennifer Carter, a resident physician who had seen him a couple of times before. After meeting with the patient, Dr. Carter came out of the exam room to explain to her attending, Dr. Suresh Mehta, that she did not see any signs of an abscess but that Mr. Gates' teeth were generally in terrible shape and he badly needed to see a dentist. She said that she explained this to her patient, but he insisted that he just needed antibiotics. She said that he was demanding them despite her best efforts and that they were at an impasse over the issue.

When Dr. Mehta entered the exam room, he saw a man in a wheelchair but noted that he did not appear to be frail or ill. Dr. Mehta extended his hand and got the bone-crushing handshake typical of sturdy older veterans. Peering into Mr. Gates' mouth, he confirmed Dr. Carter's findings: lots of severe tooth decay and inflamed gums but nothing red hot, no signs of an abscess. Despite his endorsement of Dr. Carter's assessment to Mr. Gates, the patient insisted that he did not need to see a dentist. At one point, when Drs. Carter and Mehta were looking up options for scheduling him in the dental clinic on the computer, Mr. Gates turned to his wife and said, "Let's just get out of here. They're no help." His wife did not budge. She said nothing.

Feeling his only option was to educate Mr. Gates, Dr. Mehta was about to give him a lecture on how antibiotics are not the answer to everything. His curiosity kicked in, however; and instead he asked a question, partially prompted by noticing that the patient's wife did not seem to be on the same page as her husband: "Why are you saying we are no help, when you can see that we are trying to help you?" There was a long pause during which Mr. Gates did not say anything. He just stared at the floor. Then his wife said, "He's afraid of needles. He won't go to the dentist because of the needles."

Dr. Mehta asked Mr. Gates how long he had been afraid of needles and why. Mr. Gates answered that it had started when he was a kid in the 1950s and got a polio shot. He said the people administering the shots reused the needles, and between injections they sterilized them in a flame. In his case, they had not waited for the needle to cool, so he got an injection with a red-hot and probably dull needle. He was sufficiently traumatized by that experience that he had avoided needles at all costs throughout adulthood, including visits to the dentist. Dr. Mehta wondered how many other poor Black kids from that era were similarly mistreated.

The conversation quickly transitioned to a frank discussion about traumatic experience and desensitization therapy as a treatment for his phobia. Mr. Gates acknowledged that he had not talked about it before and that no one had asked. The poor state of his mouth was a testament to a lifetime of fearing and avoiding preventive dental care. Perhaps most importantly, the tone of the interaction changed dramatically. Mr. Gates dropped his request for antibiotics, and his bitterness about not being helped dissipated.

ANOTHER REASON TO CONTEXTUALIZE CARE: LOWER COSTS

Not only are contextual errors deleterious to patient health, but they also may drive up costs, through two mechanisms: first, by resulting in the need for additional medical care and, second, by leading to unnecessary tests and treatment.

The case of Ms. Garcia's multiple ED visits because of a failure of the care team to identify and resolve her transportation situation is an example of the former. Had her situation been addressed at the first opportunity to do so, she would have had just one ED visit and hospitalization instead of four. The cost of those three unnecessary ED visits is a conservative measure of the cost of the contextual error. It does not take into account downstream costs related to lost productivity or follow-up care.

The second mechanism is illustrated with the case of Bette Wilson, who at age 59 was living with hypertension, diabetes, overweight, and recent shortness of breath and fatigue.[6] The resident, Dr. Patrick Gideon, who took the medical history and conducted the initial exam related to the supervising attending that the symptoms had worsened over the last 8 months and were relieved with rest. He also mentioned that she had smoked a pack of cigarettes a day for 10 years when she was in her twenties and thirties. In light of all these risk factors, Dr. Gideon thought he needed to determine if she had heart disease, emphysema, asthma, congestive heart failure, hypothyroidism, or chronic pulmonary emboli. He ticked off a list of imaging studies and blood tests he planned to order. As the attending headed toward the exam room to meet the patient, it was hard to disagree with the proposed plan, which seemed prudent, albeit extensive, given that it would require cardiac ultrasound, CT scanning, and nuclear imaging.

Entering the exam room, the attending physician encountered a soft-spoken woman with a gentle handshake and polite smile. Ms. Wilson recalled long-standing efforts to improve her health, including her success at quitting smoking 25 years ago, followed by less success controlling her weight until quite recently. She described embarking on an exercise program with a friend a couple of years ago and how she had begun to feel much better after losing considerable weight and becoming quite fit. She had come to enjoy shopping on foot rather than driving everywhere, was generally in a better mood, and had stopped feeling short of breath or fatigued when she exerted herself. Unfortunately, however, the gains she had made were recently lost when her friend and exercise buddy left town to care for a grandchild in another state following a daughter's divorce. Ms. Wilson acknowledged that she had returned to her sedentary ways, and with that regression, her excess weight had returned, as had her prior signs and symptoms of being out of shape.

With a few questions, the attending confirmed that the disappearance followed by reappearance of her symptoms coincided with initiation and disengagement from the long walks and activities at a fitness center that Ms. Wilson had participated in for about a year. The context for her clinical presentation was a set of specific life circumstances related to her social support, emotional state, and consequent health behaviors. They discussed several options for finding exercise buddies and agreed that Ms. Wilson would return in a few weeks to provide an update on her plan. Much expense, inconvenience, and a possible cascade of testing leading to more and increasingly invasive and costly testing were averted.

CONTEXTUALIZING CARE: WHAT DOES IT TAKE?

Health-care providers like lists because they are useful tools for remembering what to think about in a particular situation. At the heart of medical training is the "differential diagnosis," or "differential," as it is often abbreviated. The differential is a list of all the various biomedical conditions that could account for a particular cluster of signs and symptoms. For instance, the differential for chest pain and shortness of breath would include myocardial infarction (heart attack), pneumonia, and an anxiety disorder, along with several more obscure conditions.

The challenge of attending to context is that everyone's life situation is at some level unique. What kinds of things are essential to know, then, about another person in order to provide appropriate care? We refer to these as "contextual factors." For Ms. Garcia, contextual factors included her ill son and the problems she was having with transportation to her appointments. While the particulars of her situation are quite specific, to reduce cognitive load for the clinician, they can be grouped into broad categories. One could think of them as, respectively, "competing responsibilities" and issues with "access to care." For Mr. Gates, a fear of needles (the contextual factor) affected his attitude toward the health-care system and his emotional state. Based on many such cases and a series of focus groups and interviews with patients and clinicians, we identified 12 broad domains of patient context (Table 1.1).[7]

We are now often asked how "contextual factors" differ from social determinants of health or, more precisely, social risk factors. The question didn't arise until those terms were widely adopted. In some instances, contextual factors and social risk factors are nearly the same. For instance, homelessness is a social risk factor for a patient with kidney stones who is instructed to drink 3 liters of fluid a day to prevent kidney stones. Because of a lack of access to bathrooms and a water supply, they may be unable to comply. For the same reasons, it would count as a contextual factor in the domain of "environment." However, there are also scenarios in which a patient might have trouble getting to the bathroom that are not social risk factors, for instance, limited mobility due to an arthritic condition or prior injury. These would count as contextual factors. In sum, patient context is all-encompassing of the challenges in patients' lives that can complicate their care, regardless of whether they are social risk factors.[8]

There is a second, more subtle but nevertheless conceptually important, distinction between the concepts of "social risk factor" and "contextual factor" other than the latter being the larger tent: Whereas social risk factors exist independent of whether the patient is managing their care despite them, contextual factors are

Table 1.1 AREAS TO CONSIDER WHEN THERE ARE CLUES THAT
A PATIENT'S CIRCUMSTANCES OR BEHAVIORS MAY NEED TO BE ADDRESSED
WHEN PLANNING THEIR CARE

1	Access to care	7	Skills, abilities, and knowledge
2	Competing responsibilities	8	Emotional state
3	Social support	9	Cultural perspective/spiritual beliefs
4	Financial situation	10	Attitude toward illness
5	Environment	11	Attitude toward health-care provider and system
6	Resources	12	Health behavior

Reprinted with permission from the Center of Innovation for Complex Chronic Healthcare Edward Hines Jr. Veterans Affairs (VA) Hospital/Jesse Brown VA Medical Center.

defined by the evidence that they are not currently able to do so. That evidence is the "contextual red flag," the clue or symptom of an underlying contextual factor that needs to be identified or diagnosed. Housing insecurity is always a social risk factor, but it's only a contextual factor when it complicates care—or evidently soon will—from the clinician's perspective. This distinction in terminology is important in understanding the clinical nature of the latter term.

Our 12 domains of patient context can be thought of as a "contextual differential" whenever patients are struggling with life challenges that are complicating their care. Life changes in any of these areas can affect a patient's ability to manage their care. Note that they fall into two distinct conceptual groups: the six domains in the left column pertain to situations "outside the boundaries of the patient's skin," meaning, that is, life circumstances, such as financial hardship including loss of health insurance. The six on the right are drivers of behavior, such as a patient's attitude toward their illness or a change in their emotional state. To encompass the latter as well as the former in our definition of "patient context," we define it as "everything that is *expressed* outside of the boundaries of a patient's skin but that is relevant to planning their care." Although Mr. Gates' phobia is wired in his brain, its expression—avoiding dental care—is the context for his attempt to obtain antibiotics for his oral condition rather than seek definitive care.

It is likely that nearly all of us have circumstances in our lives that have implications for our health care; some of the time we are personally aware of what those contextual issues are. For instance, if we have lost the ability to pay for medication that is not covered by our health plan, we know that to be a problem. We may be ashamed, however, to mention it to our doctor. In other instances, we are not prepared to acknowledge a problem, even when it may be obvious to others who are close to us. Although Mr. Gates was not ready to volunteer the information about his underlying trauma and phobia with needles, his wife knew why he was insisting on antibiotics when what he really needed was a dentist. Finally, there are times when we are not hiding anything but are simply not aware that our care team could resolve or, at least, mitigate challenges we are facing. That was the case for Ms. Garcia, who knew what she needed to do for her grandson but did not appreciate that her dialysis could be relocated to resolve her transportation difficulties.

Because patients find it difficult to connect the dots between their health-care needs and their life context on their own, they need a close collaboration with their physician. Although there is much that an astute patient can do to alert a clinician to the relevance of context to care, it is fundamentally the physician's job to understand the need for such collaboration and consistently to take the initiative to ensure that it happens. Imagine an elderly relative or friend who begins to decline because of changes caused by early Alzheimer's disease. If they have been living independently, the deterioration may undermine their ability to take their medications. If they have diabetes, their blood sugars may become critically elevated, or if they are confused enough to take too much medication, danger-ously low. It is unrealistic to expect them to recognize that their confusion is causing their diabetes to get out of control. That is the doctor's job.

When doctors are not thinking broadly about context when considering why a disease may be getting worse, they are by default thinking narrowly about the disease process as a biomedical problem. Their focus is on the physiology exclu-sive of the surrounding context. For instance, type 2 diabetes—the most common type—often naturally progresses as patients get older because of changes that occur in the responsiveness of bodily tissues to insulin. The management of pro-gressive diabetes often involves overcoming progressive insulin "insensitivity" with additional medication. Although it is true that diabetes progresses in most patients, it is also true that there are other reasons for worsening control besides age and that considering them requires looking beyond the disease to the broader context. A clinician who thinks contextually is not doing so at the expense of thinking about the physiology but in addition to it. That breadth of thinking is re-flected in a broader differential that includes the contextual domains. The clinician who considers the domain of "skills and abilities," for instance, will look for and find deficits on cognitive testing suggesting that a new diagnosis—dementia—has emerged and must be addressed both as a biomedical problem and as a key part of the context of the patient's worsening management of their diabetes.

What does it take to think contextually? Is medical education simply failing to teach students to consider a broader differential when they evaluate disease, one that includes domains of context? That is likely a part of it, but the following anec-dote related by a late colleague, Dr. Simon Auster, about his experience observing a second-year medical student learning to interview a patient suggests there is a more fundamental problem—that current practices in medical education can make it worse:

The patient was a 62-year-old man, hospitalized for the past week, who had been recruited the previous day to meet for a practice interview. At the time he seemed in good spirits and expressed eagerness to assist. However, when we arrived that morning, he seemed distracted. As the student began to question him he responded tersely and with little interest. The student nevertheless forged ahead, trying to make his way through each compo-nent of a medical history. As the student struggled, the atmosphere in the room became increasingly oppressive. I finally considered it imperative to intervene: "Mr. Jones, you seem very upset. Is there something bothering you?" The patient explained that he was told the evening before that he would be discharged that afternoon, and he had arranged for a friend to take him home; but shortly before we arrived, he learned he would have to stay at least another day. He felt some urgency about notifying his friend who would have to leave work early to get to the hospital on time, and he had not yet been able to leave a message or reach him despite trying several numbers. However, he did not want to break his commitment to meet with the student. I said that reaching his friend was the more urgent need and that other arrangements could be made for the student. The patient's tense demeanor at once dissolved. He shook our hands as we left and reached for his phone.

As soon as we left the room the student looked at me in amazement and exclaimed "Wow. How did you do that? I tried so hard to connect with him and you knew what to say immediately." I replied, "If he had been your friend looking that upset, wouldn't you have asked him the same question?" As if a light bulb had suddenly gone on, the student exclaimed, "You mean you talk to patients like you talk to people?"

The student's genuine surprise reveals a problem that extends well beyond this student and this story. Something is missing, not only in the lists of things budding physicians are taught to ask about but in their conception of their relationship to the person they come to think of as a "patient." The patient is perceived as someone upon whom a set of tasks must be efficiently completed, rather than as a person with whom one seeks to engage with a sense of shared humanity. Simply broadening that list of tasks to include interrogating patients about their life situation is not the solution. If there is anything surprising to us about this anecdote, it is the student's candor about his revelation. Most would not be so honest or self-aware. A change in mindset is needed.

CONTEXTUALIZING CARE: FROM CHECKLISTS TO ENGAGEMENT

To engage is to connect with another person rather than just elicit and give information. The clinician who is able to engage will naturally and rapidly identify and address relevant context (i.e., contextualize care). Consider, for instance, the evaluation of a patient who passively wanted to end his own life. One well-trained resident, Dr. Sheila Bentham, knew to ask a series of questions about suicidal thoughts and plans when her patient, Mr. Beasly, commented that he had stopped taking all his medication because he "might just end it all." She asked him if he had other plans for ending his life, including whether he kept a gun in the home; he said he did not. Nevertheless, Dr. Bentham was understandably concerned and shared with her attending supervisor, Dr. Creager, that perhaps they should refer the patient to psychiatry for an immediate and more comprehensive evaluation. Dr. Bentham had completed a set of tasks yielding some useful information but did not know how to engage with Mr. Beasly.

As Dr. Creager entered the exam room he offered Mr. Beasly a gentle fist bump instead of a handshake, explaining that he was a guitarist and trying to protect his slightly arthritic hands—something he did with all his patients. Mr. Beasly smiled, saying, "That's cool. I understand." Dr. Creager seated himself on the exam table so that he could face Mr. Beasly, who was in a chair near the desk where the resident sat at a computer. Dr. Creager began, "Mr. Beasly, I understand you have been feeling down and are not taking your medications. Is that correct? Tell me what's going on." In the dialogue that followed, Dr. Creager learned about Mr. Beasly's decades of struggle with post-traumatic stress disorder (PTSD) and episodic depression dating back to his service in Vietnam in the late 1960s and early 1970s. He learned that Mr. Beasly also had a successful 30-year marriage with a wife he was comfortable confiding in. In fact, he'd promised her he'd restart his medications. Mr. Beasly had acquired a lot of skills in self-care, including avoiding PTSD triggers such as being on buses, in tunnels ("reminds me of chasing after Viet Cong in their sandals in black dark tunnels in Saigon," he said with a shudder), or in crowded public places alone, where flashbacks and intense paranoia were easily triggered. At one point during the conversation, when Mr. Beasly was relating his struggles with claustrophobia, he pointed toward the shut door and said, "Being in small rooms like this with the doors closed can freak me out." Dr. Creager interjected, "Would you like me to open the door a crack for you?" Mr. Beasly replied, "No, that's not necessary. I am feeling cared for now as you all have your attention on my health, so I'm not feeling at all like I need to get out of here. I'm feeling pretty good." During the encounter, which lasted about 7 minutes, Dr. Creager felt a connection with Mr. Beasly as well as a sense of pleasure and relief at the resilience of a man he was coming to appreciate. After asking a few more questions to see if Mr. Beasly had any tendencies toward impulsive self-destructive behavior—and determining he did not—he felt comfortable with a plan that Mr. Beasly would restart an antidepressant that had worked in the past, follow up with Dr. Bentham and himself in a couple of weeks, and call them sooner if he had any concerns. Mr. Beasly, who had not seen a physician in some time, seemed appreciative and relaxed as he headed out to the waiting area to schedule his next appointment.

After Mr. Beasly had left, Dr. Creager asked Dr. Bentham what she had learned during the encounter. Dr. Bentham thought for a moment and said, "There were some questions you asked that I had not thought of and should have known to consider. Also, I liked the way you offered to open the door when he said he had claustrophobia." Pushing a bit further, Dr. Creager said, "That's good . . . but I'm wondering did you get any sense of the man during my discussions with him that you found helpful?" Dr. Bentham looked somewhat puzzled and unsure of what to say. Dr. Creager followed gently with "Sheila, do you have an idea of what it is I am asking?" "No, I'm not sure," she replied. Dr. Creager went on to share his impressions of Mr. Beasly as someone who had strong social support, who knew himself well, and who was capable of connecting with other people. Because of these qualities, Dr. Creager related, he did not seem in danger of committing a violent act either to himself or to others. Although each of these observations was the product of a question Dr. Creager had asked, there had been no checklist. It had started with a warm greeting, followed by two people sitting together to have a caring conversation. The encounter had felt satisfying to Dr. Creager and nourishing. For Mr. Beasly, it felt healing. And a contextually appropriate care plan had emerged from the engaged interaction.

RESEARCH ON CONTEXTUALIZATION OF CARE: FROM ANECDOTE TO SYSTEMATIC STUDY

These are true stories (although we have changed the names of the patients and physicians). We find these accounts that illustrate the importance of contextualizing care to prevent contextual errors compelling. But we are researchers, and individual anecdotes are not proof of a generalized phenomenon, nor do they document the scope and magnitude of what we observed. When we started this work, we considered the idea that contextualizing care leads to better outcomes to be a hypothesis. It is a possible explanation for why so many patients do not benefit from treatments that have been demonstrated in studies to be effective. Although each example of the adverse impact of inattention to context builds a case for the importance of contextualizing care, one cannot draw strong conclusions from anecdotes.

In considering how to test our hypothesis, we realized we would have to ask and answer a couple of questions: First, how could we measure attention to relevant patient context? To do so we would need a precise definition of "relevant patient context" and a strategy for deciding whether the clinician had attended to it (and how that would be defined). Whatever definition we settled upon would require measurement tools and strategies, and those tools and strategies would need to be both valid and reliable, meaning that they were measuring what they were supposed to be measuring and that they could be counted on to deliver the same results regardless of when or by whom the measures were employed. And second, we needed a definition of a "good" versus a "bad" outcome of contextualizing (or not contextualizing) a care plan that is clinically meaningful and can be applied to predict future outcomes, rather than only in hindsight.

With tools like these, we would be able to explore the following foundational questions about clinician attention (and inattention) to patient context:

1. When a contextual factor is present, how often do physicians overlook or disregard it in their care plan, when there is a contextual red flag (i.e., a clue to its presence) or when the patient self-discloses the factor? In other words, how prone are physicians to make a contextual error when presented with an opportunity to do so?
2. In what proportion of encounters does care hinge on identifying and addressing relevant patient context?
3. What are the variations across different groups of patients with respect to the distribution of contextual factors (i.e., the 12 domains of patient context) that are complicating their ability to manage their care?
4. What are the implications for patient health-care outcomes if contextually relevant information is or is not addressed in care plans?
5. If contextualizing care does, in fact, lead to better outcomes, are there effective interventions that improve clinician attention to patient context in care planning? Specifically, is it possible to acculturate, train, and/

or nudge physicians to respond to patient context with curiosity and engagement rather than assumptions or inattention?

6. Health care is a substantial expense for both the patient and society, and policymakers are concerned not only with quality of care but the cost and value of that care. What are the cost implications of attending or not attending to context?

In the following chapters we describe the tools we employed to address these questions and what we learned—starting with the first of them in Chapter 2.

KEY POINTS

- A contextual error occurs when clinicians overlook or disregard clues that a patient is struggling with a life challenge that is complicating care.
- Contextual errors are prevented by contextualizing care, which is the process of recognizing clues that patients are struggling with life challenges that are complicating their care, identifying the underlying contextual factors (which can be grouped into 12 broad domains), and then attempting to customize the care plan so that it is adapted to the individual's specific circumstances and needs.
- Physicians pay attention to biomedical information and discount contextual information, even when the latter is just as important to achieving an effective care plan. Both psychology (the FAE) and the narrow focus of medical training help explain why physicians are often blind to context, resulting in contextual errors.
- Contextualizing care becomes a natural part of clinical practice when physicians openly and fully engage with their patients, which is typically experienced as a sense of shared humanity.

NOTES

1. Livingstone R. (1946, November). Education for the modern world. The Atlantic, 75–79.
2. Merriam-Webster. Definition of biomedical. https://www.merriam-webster.com/dictionary/biomedical. Last accessed August 14, 2022.
3. Cambridge Dictionary. Definition of context. https://dictionary.cambridge.org/us/dictionary/english/context. Last accessed August 14, 2022.
4. Weiner SJ. What is patient (life) context?: an introduction to contextualizing care (video #1 in series). https://youtu.be/dSa67tHtSkw. Last accessed August 14, 2022.
5. Ross L. The intuitive psychologist and his shortcomings: distortions in the attribution process. Adv Exp Social Psychol. 1977;10:173–220.
6. Weiner SJ. When "something is missing" from the resident's presentation. Acad Med. 2004;79(1):101.

7. Binns-Calvey AE, Malhiot A, Kostovich CT, et al. Validating domains of contextual factors essential to preventing contextual errors: a qualitative study conducted at Chicago area Veterans Health Administration sites. Acad Med. 2017;92(9):1287–1293.

8. Weiner SJ. Patient context and SDOH: how are they similar and different? Contextualizing care: fireside chat series (video #6). YouTube, n.d. https://youtu.be/xGc7T_J5b70. Last accessed August 14, 2022.

2

Measuring the Problem

"Doctor, things have been tough since I lost my job."
"I'm sorry to hear that. Do you have any allergies?"
—*Transcript of hidden audio recording*
between an undercover actor and a doctor

In this chapter we describe why contextual errors are missed by current methods for identifying error and illustrate how they can be identified and measured. A useful place to start is by reviewing briefly how medical errors have been defined and identified generally. A National Academy of Medicine report issued in 2000, *To Err is Human: Building a Safer Health System*, first drew national attention to the consequence of medical error, highlighting studies showing that 44,000–98,000 Americans die each year due to these errors—more than from car accidents, breast cancer, or AIDS.[1] These errors were deemed largely preventable through improved systems of prescribing and double-checking. More recent studies indicate the number may be quite a bit lower—22,000 (3.1% of inpatient deaths).[2] These differences reflect alternate approaches to determining whether a death can be attributed to a particular error. Throughout, however, there has been a consistent definition of what constitutes an error.

The definition is based on the work of psychologist James Reason, detailed in his book *Human Error*.[3] "Error" is "the failure of a planned action to be completed as intended (i.e., error of execution) or the use of a wrong plan to achieve an aim (i.e., error of planning)." In health care, the term "error of planning" refers to a decision-making error such as the failure to prescribe a correct plan of care because of either an incorrect diagnosis or an incorrect treatment plan for a correct diagnosis. The term "error of execution" refers to mistakes that occur during the delivery of care, including accidentally giving the wrong medication or the wrong dosage of the right medication or operating on the wrong limb. Various types of errors are often descriptively classified as diagnostic, treatment, medication, dosing, and surgical site, etc.

For the most part, medical errors have been identified by reviewing records of care. For instance, one can see that a physician's diagnosis is incompatible with a laboratory finding or that a medication administered is not the same as what was ordered, and so on. Because the human body is resilient—or because they are caught early and corrected—these errors may not cause harm. Regardless, they leave a footprint in the medical record, such that they can be tracked and their frequency measured.

By contrast, contextual errors are comparatively invisible. No laboratory value will tell you that a physician overlooked Ms. Garcia's transportation problem, although the lack of transportation may be largely responsible for the laboratory abnormalities. In fact, based on a chart review alone, it often appears that the patient received appropriate care because the context surrounding the clinical presentation is missing. Nevertheless, these lapses in care are as much errors per the definition as those readily evident during medical record reviews: Sending Ms. Garcia home without addressing her transportation needs was certainly "the wrong plan to achieve an aim" if the aim is to prevent the life-threatening abnormalities that keep bringing her back to the emergency department. Hence, contextual errors are a subtype of medical error—specifically an error of planning—that falls below the radar that is used to identify medical error.

CONTEXTUAL ERROR: THE HIDDEN SIDE OF MEDICAL ERROR

Once it became clear to us that contextual errors are missed using current measures we had to get creative about ways to detect them. So how does one identify a contextual error? Consider a man in his seventies that one of us helped care for while he was evaluated in the hospital for unexplained weight loss. Concerned about cancer, a doctor ordered a battery of tests to assess the likelihood and extent of malignancy. However, the underlying cause was not cancer but lack of food. The patient had dropped several hints that he was food-insecure and struggling with homelessness, including a comment that he "no longer has family in the area" in response to a question about what he has been eating. No one followed up to get more specific details about his cryptic response. Ordering a cancer workup instead of addressing the circumstances causing the patient's weight loss constituted "a plan of care that is inappropriate because of a failure to take into account relevant patient context" (i.e., a contextual error).

This contextual error, however, would not have been discernable using standard methods for identifying medical errors via chart review. The fundamental problem is that medical records do not show what the physician misses. If the physician did not notice or explore the patient's comment about no longer having family in the area, one of several clues that he is alone and hungry, they would not have recorded it in the chart. If we review that chart, we will see a physician make what looks like correct decisions about workup and treatment based on the medical history and the physical exam they conducted and recorded. The problem is that we don't know the truth—which is that the patient is struggling with homelessness, food insecurity, and ultimately weight loss due to malnutrition. That's the missing context. From the chart alone, there is no way to see that the context was overlooked, resulting in a contextual error—an inappropriate plan of care.

UNANNOUNCED STANDARDIZED PATIENTS: CREATING THE CONTEXT

One way to know if clinicians overlook context is to train actors to work as undercover patients portraying scripted cases in which life context is clinically relevant to appropriate care planning and then see how often physicians provide contextualized care. We adopted this approach by employing unannounced standardized patients (USPs).

A USP is a specific type of standardized patient (SP). SPs are individuals trained to consistently portray a patient with a medical problem or seeking routine care. Nearly all medical schools now use SPs to help train and test doctors. In addition to portraying a patient presentation, SPs are often trained to provide immediate feedback to students about their performance. SPs are also an important method for assessing competence. Many schools include SPs as part of their examinations, with scores based on ratings by faculty observers as well as by the SPs themselves.

Because they are standardized, SPs are ideal for assessing and comparing clinicians' clinical competencies. Every physician seeing the same SP has access to the same facts and opportunity to ask the same questions. This enables an "apples-to-apples" comparison of how physicians perform under the same conditions. It also creates ideal conditions for assessing contextual error and contextualization of care. Just as one can design a case for an SP in which actors are trained to drop clues or respond to questions about depression or tobacco use or nearly any clinical syndrome, they can also be trained to provide contextual red flags with a statement like "Boy it's been tough since I lost my job" while presenting with evidence that they have lost control of a chronic condition treated with a costly medication. In other words, patient context can be embedded into SP cases.

A limitation of SPs is the *Hawthorne effect*, in which those assessed alter their behavior because they are aware they are being observed. In medical schools, students know when they are examining an SP. Their attention is heightened, and they make efforts to show their best performance. In contrast, USPs are SPs who present to a real practice, pretending to be a real patient. At the time the doctor examines the USP, they have every reason to believe that the USP is a real patient seeking care—so we have every reason to believe that the doctor's performance is typical of what they do when seeing real patients. Hence, the introduction of contextual red flags and contextual factors into USP cases enables an authentic assessment of physician attention to patient context in actual practice.

Other terms used for USPs include "mystery patients" and "secret shoppers." Those terms are easier to say but refer to trained evaluators who report back primarily on customer service measures such as how easy it is to find the clinic, how long they had to wait to be seen, and other drivers of customer satisfaction—just like secret shoppers visiting retail stores. They do not generally assess actual delivery of care. USPs, in contrast, are standardized and "behind the curtain"—they directly observe physicians conducting medical visits.

Prior to our work, a few researchers had used USPs for studies, but the numbers of undercover visits were relatively few because the elaborate subterfuge needed to convince doctors across a wide number of practices that they are seeing real patients, not actors in disguise, is daunting. In order to get USPs into doctors' offices one has to create fake medical records, set up fake insurance information, and train actors both to keep to a script and to adapt rapidly in response to the doctors, nurses, and medical office staff. Finally, one must first gain the trust and support of the physicians involved so that they are willing to allow themselves to be fooled.

Despite the hurdles, however, it became evident to us that USPs provide an unfiltered look at how physicians perform at their jobs when they think no one is watching. To apply them to our work, however, we needed to adapt them to the study of physician attention to patient context. Specifically, how should these undercover visits be structured to collect reliable information about physicians' attention to patient context? And what should we measure? These questions brought us together—a primary care physician and a cognitive psychologist trained in the study of medical decision-making and research design—and led us into an extensive dialogue about a variety of strategies for evaluating and measuring physician attention to patient contextual information when that attention is critical to proper care. Talking together, we became excited to go beyond the many reports showing that doctors miss psychosocial issues. We set about creating an experimental system to provide the scientific evidence that was missing from previous studies. We would need to isolate and quantify (translate into numbers what had been anecdotal stories) the size of the problem so that it could be systematically analyzed. We came to USPs as a last resort, knowing how difficult it would be to send actors to visit large numbers of doctors; but we realized it was the only way to get the evidence we needed. That decision was a critical turning point in our research.

FAKE PATIENTS + REAL DOCTORS = NEW INSIGHTS

We were not the first to recognize the benefits of USPs. One of the first published reports describing an incognito patient study was "On Being Sane in Insane Places," by D. L. Rosenhan in 1973.[4] Three women and five men visited hospitals pretending to hear voices in their heads in order to get admitted to psychiatric wards. Once Rosenhan's "pseudopatients" were admitted, they stopped reporting voices. Nearly all were admitted with a diagnosis of schizophrenia and retained for 1–7 weeks, eventually being discharged with a diagnosis of "schizophrenia in remission"—the psychiatrists never recognized that the "patients" were surprisingly asymptomatic. (Interestingly, many actual patients did.)

In another study, between 2000 and 2002, a team of researchers working for the US Department of Veterans Affairs in California employed USPs to learn how accurately physicians record patient histories, physical exams, diagnoses, and treatment plans in the medical record. They sent actors to visit each of 20 physicians eight times, presenting different common complaints. The actors completed checklists of about 30 items, each based on guidelines and expert panels that inform good clinical practice. The researchers obtained the medical records of the visits and compared them to the checklists.

The medical record did not accurately represent what actually occurred during the medical encounter. Not only did physicians fail to record 14% of what they appropriately did but they also regularly documented tasks they had not performed (but should have). Physicians failed to report preventive care services delivered (e.g., tobacco cessation counseling) and, conversely, reported that they had performed physical examination procedures, made diagnoses, and, to a lesser extent, asked about medical history and planned treatments when, in fact, they had not. Overall, nearly one in five tasks that they recorded they actually had not done.[5,6,7,8,9] In another study, the same researchers demonstrated that SP checklists were highly accurate when compared with covert audio recordings of the encounters. These studies established USPs as a "gold standard" for finding out what physicians actually do during a medical encounter, both correctly and incorrectly.

USP visits seemed to us the perfect method for studying contextual errors. But to demonstrate that doctors make contextual errors, we would need our patients to show up with problems that gave the doctors a chance to explore potential contextual complications; and we had to know that those complications, if not explored and properly addressed in the treatment plan, would result in important mistakes in care. In addition, we wanted to concurrently assess their tendency to make more conventional biomedical errors to give us insight into the relative frequency of these two types of errors. To achieve these aims required an extensive process of staged case design—starting with an uncomplicated version of each case where providing appropriate care should be straightforward and then adding versions with opportunities to make biomedical, contextual, or both types of errors.

As a first step, we outlined four basic patient presentations with relatively straightforward problems. Consider Mr. James, a 42-year-old nonsmoking man who comes to see his physician about persistent breathing problems that he believes are related to his asthma. He reports that he was diagnosed with asthma as a child but rarely had problems until about 5 years ago, when he began to experience more frequent occurrences of shortness of breath and wheezing. These episodes, which occur every few days, are relieved with the use of an albuterol inhaler. He and his wife now have three young children, ages 5, 3, and 2 years, who often have colds that get passed around the family. A physician recently ordered pulmonary function tests for Mr. James, which confirmed that he has asthma. Mr. James reports that he was told he would "need one of the steroid medications" and was prescribed the latest brand-name controller inhaler, which he is to use every morning and evening regardless of whether he is experiencing symptoms. He reports that this has helped but that he is still periodically having problems with wheezing. A straightforward explanation for this problem is that his new inhaler is not sufficient to control his asthma. The usual solution would be either to increase the dose of steroids or to add another controller medication, such as Serevent° (salmeterol) or Singulair° (montelukast). (We mention brand names only as examples when we think they might be familiar, with the generic drug name in parentheses after the brand name. We are not recommending any particular brand of any drug.)

Our other basic patient presentations included Ms. Collas (a 47-year-old woman preparing for hip replacement surgery who is found to have high blood pressure), Mr. Davis (a 59-year-old man with diabetes who has been feeling faint after his previous physician increased his insulin dose), and Mr. Garrison (a 72-year-old former smoker who has been losing weight). As with Mr. James, there are evidence-based practices for each of these scenarios if no additional information contradicts them: Ms. Collas' blood pressure should be controlled prior to surgery (usually with medication), Mr. Davis needs his diet or his insulin dose modified, and Mr. Garrison needs a workup for cancer, especially lung cancer.

Next, we took those basic problems and added two different kinds of complications. The first was a medical complication: The patient could have another disease or condition that has similar major symptoms but that can be distinguished by additional symptoms the patient would mention during the visit if asked. We chose complications that required the physician to make a different treatment decision than in the basic version of the case. For Mr. James, for example, our medical complication was acid reflux, which also can cause wheezing but is treated with acid-suppressing medication rather than just asthma controller medications.

The second kind of complication was a contextual complication: The patient's life context could make the standard treatment for the basic problem just as wrong as it would be for a medical complication. For Mr. James, our contextual complication was that he had lost his job and health insurance, could no longer afford to pay for his controller medication, and was stretching it by using it only when he was having symptoms, rather than daily. Again, when this complication was present, the actor would reveal the additional information only if asked. Increasing his controller medications or prescribing additional medication would not help Mr. James get better. Rather, appropriate care would require addressing the cost issue by, for instance, switching his medication to a less costly generic.

Our study design intentionally created a parity between biomedical and contextual information, meaning that overlooking either would result in a care plan that was inappropriate. Just as it is not helpful to prescribe more asthma medication to a patient whose symptoms are due to untreated acid reflux, it is not helpful to prescribe more asthma medication that they can't afford. This format obviated the problem of skeptics saying "Well, the reason we didn't delve into the lives of these patients is that we just didn't have time and needed to prioritize." In our cases the contextual information was no less relevant than the biomedical information to planning effective care.

While this approach to case construction may seem contrived, it actually replicates what medical practice is really like. In real life doctors elicit a lot of unfiltered information from patients and then have to figure out what is significant. Some clues, if pursued, lead to important diagnoses, while others turn out to be dead ends. Hence, whenever our SPs acted out these cases, we trained them to insert both biomedical and contextual red flags (i.e., clues that the situation might have a medical or contextual complication) in all variants of a case. For example, an actor playing Mr. James would always mention, "Sometimes I wake up wheezing or coughing at night" (wheezing when lying down after meals is characteristic of reflux disease) and that "Things have been tough since I lost my job," regardless of whether they were portraying a variant of a case where these clues would turn out to be relevant to planning the patient's care.

In choosing this type of case design, we were adopting what experimental researchers call a 2 × 2 factorial design, combining the presence or absence of the two sets of complications to create four versions of each of the four patient cases (Table 2.1). Superficially, the four variants for each case seemed the same since the actor presented with the same narrative and always dropped the same clues. What varied was what happened next: If the doctor explored a clue and the version included that clue's complication, the actor would respond positively and confirm additional symptoms or contextual factors. If the doctor explored a clue and the version did not include that clue's complication, the actor would deny additional symptoms or contextual factors. So, Mr. James would always mention wheezing at night. In the medically complicated versions, if the physician asked for further information about that, Mr. James would reveal other symptoms of reflux; but if Mr. James was presenting a version that was not medically complicated, he would deny other symptoms (and indicate that his wheezing was not any more frequent at night than in the daytime). Mr. James would always mention losing his job, but if the physician asked about that, he would discuss losing health insurance (and not taking his medication regularly) only in the contextually complicated

Table 2.1 A FACTORIAL DESIGN FOR STUDYING CONTEXTUAL ERROR WITH UNANNOUNCED STANDARDIZED PATIENTS

		Medical Complication (e.g., acid reflux)	
		No	Yes
Contextual complication (e.g., job loss)	No	Basic version	Medically complicated version
	Yes	Contextually complicated version	Doubly complicated version

versions. In the versions that were not contextually complicated, Mr. James would say that he was still covered under his wife's health insurance (and using his controller medications every day). (A video explanation of our methods, employing several of our actors role-playing both patients and doctor, is available at http://www.youtube.com/watch?v=c4pYHLtvSUg.)

Before using the cases in our research, we wanted to confirm that all four versions of each case were a valid measure of a physician's competence at using relevant information to arrive at an appropriate plan of care. In particular, we wanted to be sure that the additional information offered by the patient in the biomedical or contextual (or combined) version of each case really warranted a change to the plan of care compared to the baseline version. As a test, we presented the cases in writing to a group of 16 board-certified physicians. Each version of each case was reviewed by four physicians. In the written cases, all the facts for each case were included; and in versions with complications, the confirmation of additional symptoms was also written out. For example, in the contextually complicated versions of Mr. James, the written case included the following paragraph:

> When asked about how and when he takes his medication, Mr. James states that he is "having trouble taking his medication regularly." When this is pursued, he reveals that he does not have health insurance coverage for medication and for the last 5 years has been often unemployed. He will acknowledge that he has been using his Pulmicort Turbuhaler only when his symptoms are bad, not daily, because he cannot afford the cost.

For each of our cases, we showed that all four board-certified physicians, when given the full written case, came up with the correct management and that the correct management was different for each version of a case.

We now had a tool that we could rely on to tell us whether physicians make important contextual errors. Everyone agreed on the right treatment for each version of each case when all the information was laid out and that the right treatment for the basic problem would be wrong for the complicated problems. But would physicians actually seeing these patients in their offices heed the contextual clues, discover the complications, and offer their patients the right treatment for their individual needs?

Finally, we added one further twist to the study design: For each script we drafted we hired two actors, one Black and one White, to play identical roles. The only difference would be their skin color. This would allow us to ascertain whether a patient's race alone influences physician error-making. We had reason to believe it might, given a growing number of studies indicating that Black patients get worse biomedical care. We wanted to see if these biases also increased the likelihood of contextual errors. A 2007 Harvard study, for instance, uncovered unconscious bias in the management of patients with coronary syndromes needing clot-busting drugs. Physicians were less likely to recommend these drugs when patients were Black.[10]

THE DOCTOR WILL SEE YOU NOW

The Department of Veterans Affairs (VA), which runs the hospitals and clinics that provide care to veterans of the US armed forces, is also an important sponsor of research on health care and health-care delivery. We obtained a grant from the VA's Health Services Research and Development Service (known as HSR&D), which is committed to improving access, quality, and cost of health care. Once we had funding, we began to work out how to send actors to doctors' offices undetected.

We identified 14 clinics, some part of the VA hospital system, some academic, some private. We contacted over a hundred physicians in these clinics and told them our plan: If they agreed to be in the study, they would have four visits from actors pretending to be patients some time during the following 2 years. We promised that each time they saw an actor, we would let them know as soon as they entered their note in the chart—typically within a day—so that they would not need to worry when that "patient" did not follow up to receive tests they had recommended to fill prescriptions. With the help of a staff member at each clinic, we created patient records for each visit, including insurance or payment information. Our grant paid for the costs of the visits, so the doctors and clinics did not lose money by seeing a USP instead of a real patient.

Whenever actors visited physicians, they carried hidden audio recorders that were turned on during the entire time they were in examination rooms. We used these recordings not only to learn about what the doctors did but also to check to be sure that the actors correctly portrayed the patient case. After each visit we collected the recording, and—with the help of our clinic staff insider—got copies of the medical record showing the doctor's diagnosis and management plan and the bill for the visit (showing any tests or procedures ordered and conducted during the visit). All three of these—the recording, the chart, and the bill—are important to understanding what did and did not happen. The recording reveals the plan as related by doctor to patient, the chart documents what the physician claims to have observed and ordered, and the bill provides evidence of the tests and procedures the clinic believes the patient received. Only the recording is incontrovertible; physicians can (and did) mis-record in the chart, and clinics can (and did) bill incorrectly.

Before we could get started, we needed the approval of the ethics review committees at each site where we enrolled physicians. These committees, called "institutional review boards" (IRBs), ensure that researchers minimize any potential harm to human research participants, that research participants are informed about what they will be asked to do, and that research participation is voluntary. Our research confused many IRBs: They were accustomed to protecting patients from physicians, but for our study they would be protecting physicians from (fake) patients. People accustomed to traditional biomedical research had trouble understanding the idea that the doctors were the subjects and the patients the observers. This confusion continued to dog us throughout the project. For instance, 2 years into the study, a routine audit resulted in a citation for a purported security breach. There is a rule that personal information about patients kept in hard-copy form must be kept in a locked file cabinet in a locked office. Our fake charts were stored in an unlocked cabinet in a locked VA office. When auditors discovered the cabinet was unlocked, we explained that the records—although they looked real—contained information that was entirely fictional, and we showed them the IRB-approved protocol to prove it. They filed a citation anyway. It took numerous e-mails, phone calls, and several meetings to resolve the confusion.

Once the IRBs grasped who the subjects were, they understandably wanted to make sure that physicians' reputations would not be harmed and that they knew what they were agreeing to do in the study. They were also concerned about the ethics of deceiving physicians at the time of the visit, albeit briefly, into thinking they were seeing a real patient. We argued that the study did not, in fact, involve deception because the physicians were fully informed about what would happen. They were, in essence, agreeing to be "tricked." In contrast, in the Rosenhan study (see above, "Fake Patients + Real Doctors = New Insights" section), the psychiatrists never knew that they would be seeing fake patients (and did not have the option to choose not to participate). IRBs do approve research involving deception, but only when the benefits clearly outweigh the risks and no other ap-proach could generate the needed information. This is a high bar to clear, but the IRBs were convinced by our argument. This simplified the process of obtaining approvals from all eight IRBs overseeing research across the numerous sites participating in the study.

Our next step was to hire and train actors. We began with actors who were working as SPs at what is now the Simulation and Integrative Learning Institute in our medical school at the University of Illinois at Chicago. These SPs had expe-rience role-playing patients to teach and test our medical students and residents. There is a big difference, however, between acting in a predictable environment like a stage or a training facility where people know you are acting and playing a role consistently with people who have no idea you are acting. The first actor–trainer we hired performed a "dry run" at one of our VA hospitals, portraying a female Air Force veteran, dressed for the part and well prepared with a narrative about her life to tell the physician. Her boyfriend in real life was a pilot, so she felt capable talking about flying. What she was not prepared for was the banter with real veterans that began in the waiting room:

"Hey, sister, what service were you in?"
"Ah, the Air Force."
"Really, so was I! What was your assignment?"
"I was a pilot."
"Hey, that's cool. I was a mechanic! Where were you posted?"
"Wright-Patterson."
"Really! I have a good buddy who was there probably about the same time as you, looking at your age. Did you know Greg James?"
"Um."

Another aspect we were unprepared for was what to do when physicians wanted to take immediate action: "I'm concerned about you. I'd like to do blood work now," "We need to get an ECG," and "Please change so that we can do a pelvic exam before you leave." USPs must stay on script in all communication related to the research but adapt constantly to the unexpected. We developed strategies to avoid invasive procedures: "Oh, I forgot to fast for the blood test, can I come back?" "I have a job interview and I'm running late, can we do the ECG another time?" "I am on my cycle; we'll have to do the pelvic another day."

Our first actor–trainer decided early on that this work was not for her. With our next hire, however, we struck gold. Amy Binns-Calvey, a professional actor, had experience as an SP, a track record as a successful playwright and producer, and, most importantly, extensive training in improvisation. Icing on the cake: Amy's dad, at 79 years old, was a US Army veteran, lifelong actor, and theater director who also joined our team as our oldest USP.

Preparing actors for what one of them called "doing a con" was just like putting on a successful play and required dress rehearsals. Amy had them practice by arranging visits to physicians who knew they were fakes, just so the actors could experience what it was like to go undercover in the doctor's office. We discussed and planned every detail of the process. The scripts showed the actors exactly what they had to say and do and where they could improvise. We created checklists to use when we reviewed the audio recordings of visits so that we would know how well the actors kept to the scripts and another set of checklists for keeping track of the doctors' responses and their final care plans. Even choosing and hiding the audio recorders was challenging. They had to be small, reliable, and acceptable to the IRBs. The VA only approved one type of recorder with a special kind of encryption that its privacy rules require. Amy and the actors discussed and rehearsed strategies for hiding the devices so that they would not be discovered during an exam. Actors often hid them in a lunch bag or an eyeglass case where the health-care staff and physician would not see them. After a few audio recorders failed or were accidentally turned off, we asked actors to carry two audio recorders—doubling the number of places the actors had to find to hide the devices. Remarkably, no one's audio recorder fell out of a pocket or bag or was otherwise discovered despite hundreds of visits.

Prior to each visit, our project manager, Gunjan Sharma, would work with an administrator to set up each actor visit, creating a fake identity in the electronic health record and, for the private facilities, fake insurance. Medical practices employed various kinds of electronic health record systems, so the procedures for creating a fake chart differed at each practice.

We also needed to develop a "cleaning up" process after each visit so that any records of our USP visits were removed. Electronic health record systems are designed to be secure—including to prevent the introduction of inaccurate data or the loss of patient records. We needed both to purposely "corrupt" each system with fake patient data and then to see to it that the patient data was removed after the visit.

No health record system was as difficult to adapt for USPs as the one employed by the VA health-care system. The VA electronic health record system was the worst for introducing fake patients precisely because at the time of the study it was the best for securely maintaining the records of real patients. A particular challenge is that it uses veterans' social security numbers as their medical record identifiers. As a result, creating a fake patient requires adding a fake social security number into a government database. At first, we made up nine-digit numbers just out of the range of real social security numbers. This worked until, by an untimely coincidence, the VA created filters to reject these numbers as typographical errors: If a clerk entered an out-of-range number, the system prompted the clerk to correct the error. We then went to public genealogy websites to find the social security numbers of deceased Americans and entered those. That worked until we entered numbers that had formerly belonged to veterans. The VA system keeps records of deceased veterans and alerts a central office when anyone attempts to create duplicate numbers. Our final and most successful strategy required comparing our lists of the social security numbers of deceased Americans against a database of all deceased veterans and removing the latter from the list we used for our USPs.

We did anticipate the risk of corrupting the central VA databases with fake data; we were quite concerned about it. All information on the care of millions of veterans is stored in these databases, and researchers regularly use them to conduct studies to advance medical knowledge by, for instance, looking at whether particular treatments lead to improved patient health. If fake patient data got mingled into the central databases, it would undermine their integrity and could jeopardize future medical research. Of course, we were introducing a very small number of fake patients compared with the millions of veterans in the database, and errors are regularly introduced in real patient data simply because people are not perfect at recording medical information; but we realized that we needed to avoid contributing to the problem. We partnered with the information technology (IT) division of the VA electronic health record office. On a planned schedule, we sent them lists of our USPs' social security numbers, and they intercepted their medical records before they could be incorporated into the VA National Patient Care Database. Developing such a level of trust and partnership with VA operations was an extensive process, and we are grateful to the people and offices who saw the value of our work for the future care of veterans and helped us overcome many barriers.

No amount of anticipatory planning could prepare our team for everything that could happen, and our actors' ingenuity and dedication were sometimes pushed to the limit. In one instance, a major storm struck at the time of a visit by a USP to a clinic. Evacuation alarms sounded, mandating that all staff and patients descend into a secure underground shelter. One of our actors was in the exam room feigning a severe degenerative condition of her hip, with a bad limp. She chose to stay in character and allowed herself to be convinced by staff members to go to the underground shelter; accompanied by another friendly patient, she had to limp all the way down to keep up the act.

KNIGHTS IN WHITE COTTON

Imagine placing yourself in a situation where at any time over a prolonged period, you may be examined and recorded in intimate conversation with an imposter for the sole purpose of studying your performance at your job. Over 80% of the physicians we approached consented to participate, a remarkable number under the circumstances. Across the wider medical community, the topic of direct covert observation has been contentious. In 2008, the Council on Ethics and Judicial Affairs (CEJA) of the American Medical Association (AMA) recommended the use of "secret shoppers" under limited conditions:

> Physicians have an ethical responsibility to engage in activities that contribute to continual improvements in patient care. One method for promoting such quality improvement is through the use of secret shopper "patients" who have been appropriately trained to provide feedback about physician performance in the clinical setting.

The AMA House of Delegates tabled the resolution, however; and CEJA withdrew it after a significant backlash, including concerns that it represented a failure to view the physician as a professional. Clearly, some doctors felt too threatened to endorse this new approach to observing the quality of their care, despite the suggestion that it might be a noble and ethical duty.

To overcome concerns, we reached out to a network of colleagues in the Chicago, Illinois, and Milwaukee, Wisconsin, internal medicine primary care practice communities, asking them to vouch for the integrity of the research to potential subjects. We sponsored lunch meetings at every site to tell doctors about the project and address their concerns. Most signed on when we assured them that their identities would not be disclosed, that the cost of caring for fake patients would be reimbursed, and that all that was expected of them was to do what they always do—take care of people—and not think about whether they were seeing a fake patient. When physicians agreed to participate, we typically waited several months before sending the first USP, giving them plenty of time to lose interest in the study.

Once the visits started, we began to collect evidence that the doctors thought they were seeing real patients. According to the study protocol, Gunjan was not to notify physicians that they'd seen a fake patient until they'd entered their note in the medical record. On occasion, physicians were slow to write their notes; and before the note was written, they became concerned that the patient had not yet had blood drawn or other lab tests. They would then call to ask about the missing information. All calls went to Gunjan. Introducing herself as a wife or sister or girlfriend provided an alibi. She might then say, for instance, that her husband had run off to pick up their daughter at day care and was planning to return to the clinic lab on his day off the following week. These explanations generally satisfied the providers, who were accustomed (unfortunately) to patients not following through on tests and did not suspect that it signaled they had seen a USP.

Once the doctor entered their note, Gunjan sent them an e-mail informing them that the patient was an actor. We asked them whether they had suspected that they had been caring for a USP. Many would say that, in hindsight, they had suspected it was a fake patient. But when we tried, instead, asking physicians to e-mail *us* when they thought they had seen a fake patient, we received e-mails about real patients. We expected this because it also happened to Rosenhan during a follow-up experiment in "On Being Sane in Insane Places." Several hospitals not involved in the original study invited him to send pseudopatients to their facility, convinced that they could tell the difference between real and fake mentally ill patients. He agreed but sent no undercover observers. All of the participating sites started reporting that they had identified the imposters—all of whom were actually real patients.

An important lesson—and an instruction we gave to all of our participating physicians—was never to assume a patient was a fake. Perhaps the only way a real patient could have been harmed in our study would have been if a doctor had called them out mistakenly as a fake. The physicians were instructed never to do so, and there were no reported incidents.

Although the project moved along smoothly for the most part at the academic and private practices, we periodically lived in fear that the VA would shut the study down at VA facilities. This may seem odd because the VA was actually funding the study. But an organization so large does not speak with one voice. The senior leadership at the time was responding to several widely publicized losses of veterans' personal information, including social security numbers, as a result of thefts of laptops and hard drives. At one VA hospital, for instance, an IT specialist lost an external hard drive containing the social security numbers of about 535,000 veterans. The VA's Office of the Inspector General was omnipresent, and directives to enhance data security seemed to consume the bureaucracy.

The first suggestion that authorities were concerned about our project came from Dr. Seth Eisen, the national director of the HSR&D, the unit that was paying for the study. He explained, apologetically, that he had been instructed to tell us we could no longer create or use fake social security numbers. This was tantamount to informing us that we would have to terminate the study. When we pointed out to him that there was no possible way that a fake patient could be harmed by disclosure of a fake social security number, Dr. Eisen agreed but said, "I think this is mainly a PR thing. The VA is just too concerned about what could come out in the press." He declined to say who was telling him we had to close shop, saying only, "They mean it."

Interestingly, after that call we never received a follow-up e-mail documenting the directive. It struck us as unusual that a senior VA official would not create the usual paper trail. Perhaps it was a friendly and informal warning, and it was up to us to decide what to do next. We decided to keep the study going.

When an e-mail did arrive, it came from the chief of staff of the Jesse Brown VA Medical Center, one of our data collection sites, with a specific order to cease the study immediately. This time we followed orders.

The VA health-care system is divided into 21 regions, known as Veterans Integrated Service Networks (VISNs). Jesse Brown, along with three other VA sites where we were collecting data, were all in VISN 12, which covers large sections of Michigan, Wisconsin, Illinois, and Indiana and includes dozens of clinics and seven medical centers. The Jesse Brown chief of staff explained that the request to close the study had come from the chief medical officer of VISN 12, Dr. Jeff Murawsky.

Dr. Murawsky's office, in a lovely brick building on the campus of Hines Hospital in Maywood, Illinois, about 10 miles west of downtown Chicago, had the classical feel of an admissions office at a small New England college. It seemed worlds away from the buzz and hum of the large bureaucratic institutions reporting to the VISN office. Our meeting with Dr. Murawsky also included Frances Weaver, PhD, director of the health services research center in VISN 12 and a coinvestigator on our USP study.

By a stroke of good fortune, we had a special connection to Dr. Murawsky. Several years earlier, before he had been promoted to VISN chief medical officer, Dr. Murawsky—Jeff, as we knew him—had been a primary care physician in one of the clinics where we did the early tests of methods for sending fake patients to VA facilities. Back then, we had been referred to Jeff as one of the doctors who knew the medical record system better than most and would be a good partner in the tests. We met a few times and arranged for several actors to visit Jeff's office undercover to see what worked. As a result, Jeff understood the project and knew why it mattered.

Jeff—or, rather, interim VISN chief medical officer Dr. Murawsky—was now sitting behind a desk, staring at the directive to shut down the study. He began by asking to review each of the levels of approval we had received: Do you have all IRB approvals? Have the facility privacy officers signed off on the project? Have all your laptops and flash drives been certified as encrypted with VA-approved software? What about HIPAA authorization? (HIPAA, the federal Health Insurance Portability and Accountability Act of 1996, mandates a set of policies for protecting the privacy of individually identifiable health information during medical treatment, billing, and research.) The list went on. We had all of the documents. Jeff thought for a moment and then explained, "My job is to make sure you are compliant with all policies and practices for the administration of your duties which, in this case, is to conduct meritorious research that has been funded and vetted by the US government and that meets all requirement of the VISN. You are compliant. You may proceed with the study. I'll let the chiefs of staff know."

Jeff's decision to overrule an order from a national office based on a thorough understanding of his role and a recognition that he had something of value to stand up for struck us all as brave. Not long thereafter, "interim" was dropped from his title, and he was named the permanent VISN 12 chief medical officer; a few years later, he was appointed from Washington to become VISN director. The VA is funny that way. On the one hand, it is a large, impersonal bureaucracy, with countless directives rushing like rapids downhill from top leadership to individual physicians and researchers. At the same time, there is a humanistic countercurrent, with people like Jeff and Seth quietly helping small boats through turbulent water.

THE PROBLEM IS REAL

By the end of the study, our actors had made 399 visits to 111 board-certified practicing physicians at 14 different offices. In 73% of the uncomplicated cases, physicians made the right diagnosis and ordered an appropriate plan of care (e.g., increasing the dosage of medication for the asthma patient). When the actors portrayed medically complicated cases, however, the rate of success fell to 38% (e.g., the asthma patient's acid reflux was missed). And when the actors portrayed contextually complicated cases, the rate of success was even lower—just 22% (e.g., the asthma patient's inability to afford their medication was not considered). That is, in over three-quarters of cases when physicians saw patients with con-textual factors, they made errors (Table 2.2). We came to call this a "biomedical bias": Physicians were more likely to look for and uncover something medically significant about a patient than something socially significant even when a social issue accounted for the medical problem, hence the high frequency of contextual errors.

About half of these errors occurred because physicians failed to probe contex-tual red flags, their performance varying according to case. We saw no significant difference in performance between physicians practicing in the VA health-care system (where many patients have contextual complications and we might expect physicians to be particularly well attuned to them) and those in private, group, or academic practice. We also saw no differences when the actor was Black compared with White.

Because these visits were audio-recorded and because physicians saw the "same" patients, we were able to look at the impact of time spent with patients on error rates, both biomedical and contextual. The findings were mixed: On the one hand, physicians who spent more time with patients were more likely to probe both kinds of red flags. For every additional minute of "face time"—time during the recording when the physician was actually present in the room—the odds that

Table 2.2 Frequency of Contextual Error Among Physicians as Measured by Unannounced Standardized Patients

		Medical Complication	
		No	Yes
Contextual complication	No	Basic problem 27% errors	Medically complicated problem 62% errors
	Yes	Contextually complicated problem 78% errors	Doubly complicated problem 91% errors

the physician would probe a medical red flag went up by 8%, and the odds that the physician would probe a contextual red flag went up by 5%. What this means is that for every 10 patients with contextual issues who are scheduled into 15-minute rather than 30-minute visits, one of them will present a contextual red flag that the physician will miss due to lack of time. As visits get shorter, physicians are more likely to overlook clues that may be essential to planning effective care.

On the other hand, we saw how more time to explore was not enough to result in better care; the doctor also needed to plan an appropriate treatment. In the medically complicated cases, when doctors probed and discovered medical complications, they planned the right treatment 31% of the time. In the contextually complicated cases, however, even when doctors probed and discovered contextual complications (i.e., contextual factors), they planned the right treatment only 20% of the time. We saw this difference in all types of practices and for both Black and White actors. Although physicians who spent more time with patients were more likely to probe red flags, more time did not lead to a greater likelihood of incorporating the results of probing into the treatment plan. Turning that around, visits in which physicians did a great job of putting together all the necessary information and planning appropriate care were not on average any longer than those in which they did not. Something about the way physicians at their best think and communicate during those visits improves care without increasing the time required to do so. We will return to this observation later in the book when we discuss ways to improve contextualized care.

We published the results of our study in the *Annals of Internal Medicine*.[11] *Annals* accompanied the paper with an editorial in which the author provided examples of contextual errors he had encountered, concluding, "How much better to learn these hard lessons from standardized patients, for both physicians and real patients, and less expensive in the long run."[12] The *Chicago Tribune* ran a front-page story with the headline, "'Mystery Patients' Help Uncover Medical Errors," which included interviews with participating physicians.[13] One of them, Dr. Eric Christoff, observed, "I see this as an opportunity. All of us have a lot to learn about how we can do our jobs better." We were invited onto talk radio shows to explain the study and its results.

Despite the brief attention to our work, interest soon waned. The work was not often cited, and others didn't attempt to replicate or advance what we had done. We considered several possible reasons: First, the concept of a "contextual error" is somewhat abstract, and the research methods we used to identify these errors were quite novel and, as a result, require considerable effort to understand. Although it's straightforward to understand the significance of a conventional medical error (e.g., giving the wrong medication for asthma), it's harder to grasp the implications of overlooking life context (e.g., giving the right treatment but not realizing that the patient won't be able to take it because of cost) even when the effect on outcomes is the same. Another reason is that carrying out this type of research is logistically very complex, as detailed above. You can't just go to a database. Rather, you have to find dozens or hundreds of physicians and one or more health systems that will support an elaborate subterfuge in the name of science.

And, finally, a third possible reason for relatively low interest was that our work was published before concerns about the social determinants of health had emerged. Our USP study came out 9 years before the National Academy of Medicine published *Integrating Social Care into the Delivery of Health Care: Moving Upstream to Improve the Nation's Health* in 2019.[14] In that report they distinguished between social factors that require community-level interventions and those where the clinician can help the patient directly. With regard to the latter, they identified two types of interventions: adjustments, in which the physician essentially comes up with a work-around (e.g., putting the patient on a less costly medication they can afford), and assistance, in which the clinician draws on available resources to help (handing out free samples of a medication if available). They linked these types of interventions back to our USP research, noting that "Health services researchers have described clinical care that incorporates an understanding of social context as 'contextualized care' (Weiner et al., 2010)."

Working with USPs also turned up some unexpected observations outside of our study aims that suggest larger problems that require further USP research to better understand. USPs provide a window into what happens within the black box of a medical visit that goes uncharted in the medical record. For instance, although our Black actors got the same care as their White counterparts playing the same scripts, they had a harder time signing in when they told clerks they were uninsured. They reported they were more likely to be told they could not be seen, even though they were presenting with exactly the same life story and presenting complaint as their White counterpart.

We also discovered idiosyncrasies of systems and providers that could disrupt the care or study process. Some doctors would take long personal phone calls during a visit, occasionally without even leaving the exam room. Others left the room when the patient changed but attended to other patients, leaving the patient in a gown for what seemed an unduly long period of time. Some physicians focused on the computer screen, entering notes, as opposed to making eye contact with the patient. Quite a few physicians focused their attention on the weight of one of our actors, even though it was not a part of his scripted problem. He wanted to talk about his asthma; they wanted to tell him that he weighed too much and needed to diet. He confessed that he found this sufficiently irritating that it made it difficult to stay on script. Another of our USPs, after providing clues that he was seriously depressed—in accordance with his script—was told by the doctor "not to go anywhere." The doctor said he would send in a mental health professional shortly to evaluate the patient and left the exam room. No one returned in his place, and after 40 minutes, the actor left. In one private office, the physician was angry that a new patient had been added to his schedule. The USP stood there awkwardly while the physician chided his office staff, saying "you know my practice is closed to new patients." Clearly, he had forgotten about the study and that he had agreed to the possibility of being audio-recorded. Finally, we occasionally uncovered billing problems. At one site we received a bill for electrocardiograms that our patients had declined. The clinic's financial office was skeptical when we told them these were fake patients who had refused the procedure—until we showed them the transcripts of the audio recordings. Only then did they acknowledge that patients were getting billed as soon as a physician ordered the test, regardless of whether the test occurred. Although our focus was on contextual care, the USP process offered a much broader view of the health-care system.

THE (ECONOMIC) COST OF CONTEXTUAL ERROR

Although we'd shown that contextual errors could actually harm patients, we did not initially look at their economic impact. Using USPs, we had shown that experienced and fully credentialed physicians make contextual errors frequently, both because they fail to probe contextual red flags and because they fail to apply what they had learned by eliciting contextual factors when they did probe. We knew from the design of the patient cases that these contextual errors would have had important health consequences had the patients been real. In health terms, these were costly errors. But what about their impact on actual costs of care?

Because we also obtained the billing records from the visits, we were in a position to ask whether these errors also cost more money. Calculating the full cost of medical care is surprisingly tricky. We focused on direct medical costs—how much it would cost to treat a correctly diagnosed medical problem. We also limited ourselves to costs that might be expected within 30 days of the visit. We did not try to consider indirect costs, such as the cost of transportation to the clinic or lost wages during illness, or long-term costs, such as the possibility that a patient might need hospitalization later as a result of ineffective care. Finally, we calculated costs based on standard Medicare reimbursement schedules, rather than on the clinic's billing charges (which include overhead, profit, and other costs that are not really medical). We were being conservative: If we had considered any of these other costs, the contextual errors we found would have been even more expensive.

To calculate the financial cost of errors, we considered three different ways a treatment plan could go wrong. First, the physician might order unnecessary care that could have been avoided if context had been properly considered. This is *overuse* of medical resources. If a patient does not have reflux disease, but a doctor prescribes an antacid anyway, that is overuse. It is easy to figure out how much overuse costs—it is the cost of the unnecessary care the patient receives. When it was clear from our case that the patient would not actually receive the unnecessary treatment—for example, when the asthma patient without health insurance was prescribed a more expensive inhaler that he also could not afford—we made the conservative choice to consider the cost of overuse to be nothing.

Second, the physician might fail to order necessary care that they would have ordered if context had been properly considered. This is *underuse* of medical resources. If a patient does have reflux disease and does not get a medication that treats it, that is underuse. It is harder to put a cost on underuse, so we again made a conservative assumption. We decided that the values of common evidence-based treatments were at least as great as their costs, or else such treatments would not be recommended. So when a physician did not order a generic inhaler for an asthmatic patient, we considered the cost of that error to be the cost of the inhaler for a month.

Third, a physician might both order an unnecessary treatment and miss a necessary treatment. We call this combination of overuse and underuse *misuse* of medical resources, and we combine the cost of the overuse and underuse to get the cost of misuse.

In this study alone, we found a total of $174,000 in avoidable costs, mostly from underuse. In comparing costs of errors in different kinds of cases, we looked at the median cost of errors. The median is the value for which half of the visits with errors had higher costs of error and half had lower. We prefer the median to the more common average (the mean) because the median is less affected by a small number of extremely costly visits.

The median cost of errors in uncomplicated cases was $164 per visit when an error occurred. In biomedically complicated cases with errors, the median cost of error was $30. But in contextually complicated cases with errors, the median cost of error was $231 per visit, which is substantially higher than in either uncomplicated or biomedically complicated visits. In doubly complicated cases, the median cost of error was $224 per visit, similar to the contextually complicated cases. Contextual errors are not only more frequent than biomedical errors but more costly when they occur (Figure 2.1). Of that $174,000 in costs of errors, almost $152,000 came from contextually or doubly complicated visits.

As noted earlier, these costs are hard to detect because the errors that cause them are often hidden. Because we had the medical records, we were able to

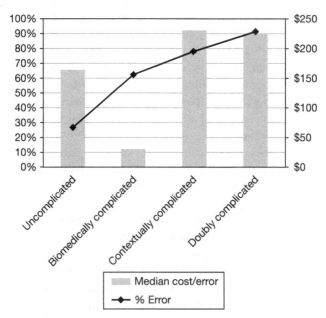

Figure 2.1 Frequency and median cost of contextual errors detected by unannounced standardized patients.

compare the true cost of errors detected in our study using the gold standard of USPs with what one could discern solely from our patients' charts. We found that no more than $8,745 of the $174,000 in avoidable costs would have been detected through medical record review (just 5%)—and these were all from non-contextual errors that physicians made in the uncomplicated cases. When a physician records a high blood pressure but fails to treat it, the error can be seen in the chart. The medical record did not help us identify contextual errors, however, because doctors cannot write what they do not observe. Physicians in our study had particular trouble identifying necessary contextual information, and so contextually complicated cases were more likely to have incorrect diagnoses and treatment plans. And the costs of these frequent errors, like the errors themselves, were not discernable from a medical record review.[15]

A limitation of this research is that we could not factor in the downstream costs of future care needs caused by contextual errors. That was, of course, because our patients were fake. Had our patient with asthma who could not afford his medication been real, how likely would he have been to require future care—including an emergency room visit or even a hospitalization—because no one figured out that he needed a less costly generic? And, more broadly, how common are such occurrences? One thing we could not discern with USPs was how often contextual errors occur in actual practice. To find that out, we would have to watch doctors with real patients, and that was our next step.

KEY POINTS

- Contextual error is a subtype of medical error because it involves the use of a wrong plan to achieve an aim.
- Contextual errors are generally not detectable from a medical record review. Detecting them requires knowing what information a patient shared during the medical encounter and whether the physician appropriately followed up.
- USPs enable researchers to study the conditions under which clinicians make contextual errors and the frequency with which the errors occur. They also enable benchmarking of contextual error rates against the better-known biomedical errors that have been previously reported.
- In the large USP study reported in this chapter, physicians made contextual errors over three-quarters of the time when they were given the opportunity to do so, a higher rate than with comparable biomedical errors.
- Surprisingly, time spent with patients was not a predictor of contextual error rates. When physicians took time to probe, identify, and address contextual factors, they made it up in other parts of the visit, perhaps by not having to discuss and order unnecessary care.
- In the study described, the costs of contextual errors were much higher than the costs of biomedical errors, even using highly conservative

methods for calculating costs. It is unknown to what extent the finding
would generalize to other clinical scenarios and settings. The findings
suggest, however, that contextual errors contribute substantially to overall
health-care costs.

NOTES

1.   Kohn LT, Corrigan JM, Donaldson MS, eds. To err is human: building a safer
     health system. Washington, DC: National Academies Press; 2000.
2.   Rodwin BA, Bilan VP, Merchant NB, et al. Rate of preventable mortality in
     hospitalized patients: a systematic review and meta-analysis. J Gen Intern Med.
     2020;35(7):2099–2106.
3.   Reason JT. Human error. Cambridge, England; New York: Cambridge University
     Press; 1990.
4.   Rosenhan DL. On being sane in insane places. Clin Soc Work J. 1974;2(4):237–256.
5.   Dresselhaus TR, Luck J, Peabody JW. The ethical problem of false positives: a pro-
     spective evaluation of physician reporting in the medical record. J Med Ethics.
     2002;28(5):291–294.
6.   Glassman PA, Luck J, O'Gara EM, Peabody JW. Using standardized patients to
     measure quality: evidence from the literature and a prospective study. Jt Comm J
     Qual Improv. 2000;26(11):644–653.
7.   Luck J, Peabody JW, Dresselhaus TR, Lee M, Glassman P. How well does chart ab-
     straction measure quality? A prospective comparison of standardized patients with
     the medical record. Am J Med. 2000;108(8):642–649.
8.   Peabody JW, Luck J, Glassman P, Dresselhaus TR, Lee M. Comparison of vignettes,
     standardized patients, and chart abstraction: a prospective validation study of 3
     methods for measuring quality. JAMA. 2000;283(13):1715–1722.
9.   Luck J, Peabody JW. Using standardised patients to measure physicians' prac-
     tice: validation study using audio recordings. BMJ. 2002;325(7366):679.
10. Green AR, Carney DR, Pallin DJ, et al. Implicit bias among physicians and its pre-
     diction of thrombolysis decisions for black and white patients. J Gen Intern Med.
     2007;22(9):1231–1238.
11. Weiner SJ, Schwartz A, Weaver F, et al. Contextual errors and failures in individualizing
     patient care: a multicenter study. Ann Intern Med. 2010;153(2):69–75.
12. LaCombe MA. Contextual errors. Ann Intern Med. 2010;153(2):126–127.
13. Graham J. (2010, July 19). "Mystery patients" help uncover medical errors. Chicago
     Tribune.
14. National Academies of Sciences Engineering, and Medicine. Integrating social care
     into the delivery of health care: moving upstream to improve the nation's health.
     Washington, DC: National Academies Press; 2019. https://doi.org/10.17226/25467.
15. Schwartz A, Weiner SJ, Weaver F, et al. Uncharted territory: measuring costs of di-
     agnostic errors outside the medical record. BMJ Qual Saf. 2012;21(11):918–924.

3

The Problem Is Everywhere

DOCTOR: "Do you want a shingles shot?"
PATIENT: "I never heard of it."
DOCTOR: "You didn't get any information from your friends?"
PATIENT: "What?"
DOCTOR: "Shingles! Shingles!"
PATIENT: "What is it?"
DOCTOR: "Chickenpox! It prevents you against chickenpox."
PATIENT: "I had chickenpox already, they say you're only supposed to get it one time."
DOCTOR: "Even then you can get chickenpox again, not chickenpox, it's called shingles. If you don't want it, I'm not going to force you."

—Transcript of hidden audio recording
between a real patient and doctor

Studying how doctors care for actual patients may seem like a step forward from studying their interactions with unannounced standardized patients (USPs), but in some respects, it was also a step back. Sending a USP portraying a script to a group of physicians is a controlled experiment. The doctors are the subjects, and what the USP is trained to say and do is the "stimulus." They present the same way to each physician. This, of course, never happens in real life as no two actual patients are exactly alike. For instance, two patients may both have diabetes, but one is older and has kidney disease. The expectations for the physicians managing their diabetes would not be quite the same. And expected outcomes would differ as well. As a result, measuring variations in quality of care requires adjusting, using statistical methods, for patient differences—a process that is quite imperfect. With USPs, in contrast, everything except the variables of interest is held constant, a characteristic that is sometimes referred to as "intrinsic risk adjustment."

Well, nearly everything else is held constant. We say "nearly" because while the USP is standardized, the clinical setting is not. While two doctors may get

Table 3.1 ADVANTAGES OF STUDYING CONTEXTUALIZATION WITH
UNANNOUNCED STANDARDIZED PATIENTS VERSUS REAL PATIENTS

Advantages of Using Unannounced Standardized Patients	Advantages of Using Real Patients
Control over case mix	Can measure frequency of various contextual factors
Control over contextual red flags and contextual factors	Can measure actual health outcomes and costs
Correct plan known in advance	Does not require creating fake charts, insurance records, etc.
Can be tailored to study performance in particular diseases, patient populations, etc.	Less expensive than unannounced standardized patients
Cannot interfere with actual care	

the same USP, one may be rushed and the other may have no time pressure. We try to account for such differences—and any others we identify—for example, by collecting data on whether physicians are running late when they see a USP and making allowances for that in our analysis. This helps us isolate the effect of a contextual factor on physicians' behavior (e.g., whether they switch patients who can't afford a medication to a less costly alternative).

So, why change our research method? For a comparison of the methods, highlighting some advantages of each, see Table 3.1. First, working with USPs was getting to be too hard. Although the Veterans Administration (VA) had let us finish our USP study, it was clear we could not do anything like it again anytime soon. We continue to advocate for a simpler process and more welcoming environment for including USP research and quality improvement both within and outside of the VA. After all, nothing compares with USPs for getting accurate information about what doctors and other staff would do when faced with a particular patient scenario.

The main reason, however, for transitioning to real patients is that doing so addresses one big limitation of working with USPs: They tell you nothing about the diversity of challenges clinicians actually face. Our entire USP study was based on how doctors handle four common clinical situations. Of course, doctors deal with many other problems besides those four. Finally, studying contextualization of care with real patients afforded us an opportunity to look at the impact of contextualization of care, or the failure thereof, on patient health-care outcomes. Having proven that physicians often make contextual errors when given the opportunity to do so, we could now address the question "Does it matter?" If patients receiving contextualized care do no better or worse than those whose care is rife with contextual errors, then who cares? Intuitively, contextualizing care should lead to better outcomes. But could we show it? By tracking the health-care outcomes of real patients whose encounters have been audio-recorded and coded for contextualization of care, we could find out.

Moving to real patients required addressing several fundamental challenges. First was the fact that, as far as we could tell, no one had ever asked real patients if they would like to covertly audio-record their visits with their doctors. How would patients respond to such an opportunity? Second, we did not know how doctors would feel about it either. Third, after satisfying both of these stakeholders, we also would have to obtain ethical approval from an institutional review board (IRB). And, fourth, we would need a method for assessing clinician performance at contextualizing care when we were no longer scripting the cases—one that would convincingly discern those interactions and resulting care plans that were contextualized from those that were not. Taking all of these factors into account, we'd need to develop a process that everyone—patients, physicians, and clinics—would support.

Whereas in our study employing USPs we recruited attending physicians as subjects, for this project we decided to enroll resident physicians instead. This was partly a matter of convenience and circumstance. Over 100 attendings had good-naturedly participated in our research for 3 years, and we did not want to wear their patience thin. Another advantage of moving on to residents is that we could enroll a large number of them from just two hospital clinics that host residency training programs, instead of having to seek out attendings at over a dozen practices. The main reason, however, was that we also wanted to see whether an educational intervention could improve contextualization of care. We discuss the findings of that part of our project in Chapter 6, where we explore the potential for educating clinicians to contextualize care.

Before writing the proposal, we informally asked residents how they would feel about being audio-recorded by their patients if they could be assured that the data would never go to their supervisor or to anyone else outside of the research team. The most common concern raised was that they thought it would be awkward to have an audio recorder sitting there while they were interacting with a patient. When we clarified that we would ask each patient to conceal the audio recorder, they thought that was reasonable. A common refrain was, "As long as I don't need to think about it and it's not on my mind, then that's fine."

We also asked patients what they thought. (Because both these clinics are at VA facilities, the patients were all veterans.) We asked them how they would feel about collecting data using a concealed audio recorder, knowing that their physicians had agreed to participate without coercion, for a study of whether we could improve the quality of care they receive. We also explained that the data would be stored on a secure VA server with the same security standards that are used to store the rest of their medical information. The main concern that came up was not wanting to risk hurting their doctors, to whom many felt loyal. Some would say, "I'm not spying on my doctor!" Most, however, said they felt fine about it as long as it could help improve care to fellow veterans.

Once we had sounded out the physicians and patients, we knew we could handle the other aspects of this project, drawing on our prior experience working with USPs. We were familiar with the various logistical challenges, legal requirements, and IRB expectations. Obtaining funding is almost always a huge hurdle, but this time we got lucky. The VA had put out a call for proposals for studies to improve care through provider education. It appeared to be one of those situations where they had some residual funds to commit before the end of the fiscal year. They wanted proposals on short notice and said that they would attempt to fund them on the first round if possible, averting the need for resubmissions. This contrasted with the excruciating process that typically is required. Our proposal for the USP study had taken three submissions, each requiring months of work, followed by months of waiting. This time, our proposal got approved in one cycle without much of a wait time. Like so many things in life, this had less to do with us and more with the context!

Once funded, the first step was to figure out who to hire for our project team. A research team typically consists of a principal investigator, coinvestigators who are career scientists or clinicians, and staff with titles such as "research assistant," "research coordinator," etc. These individuals may be aspiring medical students, professionals with a bachelor's or master's degree in a relevant discipline, or people just looking for an interesting job. They are paid from grant funding, which is inherently time-limited.

We knew two of our team would be Gunjan Sharma and Amy Binns-Calvey. Gunjan had become our expert at working with practices not only to schedule USP visits but to obtain medical records after the visit, which we knew would be just as important with real patients. Amy, of course, was our USP trainer and coordinator. Both had spent time listening to visit recordings and coding them in our USP studies, and both were eager to develop an approach to coding actual visits. We also knew, however, that we would need more people, both for coding and for recruiting patients to participate. We needed individuals who were highly adaptive and could fulfill a variety of atypical roles requiring substantial improvisation. They would spend several days each week in noisy clinics approaching veterans to explain our project and ask if they would carry concealed audio recorders into their appointments. Over a period of several years they would listen to thousands of hours of audio recordings, systematically developing a coding system under our supervision but with much of the innovative thinking falling to them. Throughout, they would learn the unique culture of the VA health-care environment and numerous complex regulations related to human subject research.

Amy, deeply involved in the Chicago acting community, introduced us to Brendan Kelly and Naomi Ashley, both of whom had theater and music backgrounds. Brendan was working at Chicago's Shedd Aquarium, where he narrated the dolphin exhibit several times a day to hundreds of screaming kids and their families. He, Amy, and a third actor also had a long-running show called *The Weird Sisters*, a wry off-color musical comedy. Brendan proved to be highly versatile. For instance, we cast him as the physician in an instructional video that we developed for the journal *Annals of Internal Medicine*, describing one of our studies. He looked the part. The work at the aquarium was insecure, so Brendan was open for a change.

Naomi is a singer–songwriter with extensive experience playing around the city. She grew up in Nebraska and came to Chicago to pursue a career in music. For several years, Naomi worked as assistant to the head of the Department of Family Medicine at the University of Illinois Chicago. Naomi, Brendan, and Amy exemplify characteristics of theater people: They are accustomed to both highbrow and lowbrow work, to functioning in an ever-changing environment, and to living with uncertainty about what will happen next. Actors may find themselves, in the span of a day, both applauded by well-heeled urban professionals after playing in *Othello* and, to make ends meet, serving those same individuals as restaurant waitstaff. It's all in a day's work.

But the main reason we hired Brendan and Naomi is because Amy recommended them. Amy's signature attribute, other than accomplishing so much without bothering to get a college degree (until we finally nudged her to do so through an online correspondence program), is her exceptional judgment. If she thought a dolphin show narrator and a singer–songwriter were the right people to help us study physician decision-making, those were the people we wanted.

Once the protocol for our study was approved by the IRBs at the two facilities where we would be conducting the research, the first step was to begin the consent process, where we would obtain permission from research subjects to include them in the study. Of course, we had two different sets of subjects: doctors and patients. We started by recruiting the former. We attended standing meetings of the residents, with the permission of their residency program director, to introduce them to our study. We explained to the residents that their participation would have no bearing on their status in their program. A perk, if they saw it that way, was that half of them would be randomized to participate in four hour-long workshops on contextualizing care, to occur in the mornings over several weeks in lieu of another educational conference they generally attend—and with fresh fruit and pastries from the Corner Bakery. Both those enrolling in our workshop and those in the control group would participate in an evaluation at the Clinical Performance Center with standardized patients, again accompanied by breakfast. Finally, all participating residents would be assessed from audio recordings collected by their patients carrying concealed recorders over the coming months. No identifiable data would leave the research team. After explaining all this at resident meetings, we handed out a clipboard for them to sign their name if they were interested in learning more.

The reference to free breakfast may seem like an unnecessary detail. In our experience, however, it is just such details that make or break million-dollar studies. Getting those Corner Bakery breakfasts covered by grant money took months of paperwork and negotiation with federal budgeting and contract offices. In general, one cannot use government money to pay for food at meetings. When it became clear to us that we just were not going to have any human subjects for research unless we fed them a decent breakfast, we knew that we had to find a workaround. It turns out that if one can document that the educational sessions can only occur during times when subjects would eat, you can seek approval to find a vendor to provide food. We got a signed legal opinion in support of our request. The next challenge was finding approved vendors for breakfast food delivery. Although we repeatedly reference Corner Bakery above, the approved vendors would periodically change without notice. Sometimes it was Corner Bakery, sometimes Cosi or Au Bon Pain, and periodically the government would refuse to pay entirely; but we managed to use some privately donated funds to fill that gap.

Working off the list of residents interested in learning more, we began to contact them to see if they formally would consent to participate. Over a 30-month
period, 139 agreed to do so. Obtaining consent from our second group of subjects,
actual patients, also began with asking about their interest. We could not, however, directly approach them, for privacy reasons. Hence, the patient recruitment
process began when a patient approached the front desk and registered for their
appointment with a clerk. The clerk was coached to mention that there was an
ongoing study underway to improve care, and if the patient wished, they could
help collect some of the information needed for research. The clerk would point
toward a member of our team, typically Brendan or Naomi, and tell the veteran to
talk with one of them if they wanted to know more.

Inviting patients to covertly audio-record their encounters with their physicians
was uncharted territory. The process didn't even have a name, so we began calling
it "patient-collected audio"—a term we still use. We realized early on that only
a minority of patients would likely be comfortable participating. No one should
feel even slightly pressured to participate. A patient either should be completely
comfortable with the idea or should not do it at all. Many of those who said "yes"
did not think it was a big deal. They casually would place the small device in a
shirt pocket or bag and often forget it was there. Following the visit, if we did
not spot them coming out of the office area, it was sometimes necessary to chase
them down the hallway to retrieve the recorder as patients absentmindedly left
with the devices in their pockets and still on. A second group of patients who also
readily consented to participate harbored the idea that they were spying. Upon
entering the exam room, they would take out the audio recorder, show it to the
doctor, and say, "Somebody out there asked me to spy on you." The residents were
good-natured about it and would typically respond with something like, "That's
no problem. That's just a research study I'm in." Despite our best efforts, we could
not find a way either to disabuse these veterans of their concern or even to identify
the concern during the consent process. Whenever they sensed any apprehension,
Naomi and Brendan advised veterans not to participate. About 40% of veterans
they talked with signed on.

As noted earlier, a major difference between sending in patients with narratives
of our own design versus sending in real patients to audio-record encounters is
that we didn't know how often there would be contextual red flags to probe and
contextual factors to address. Whereas every one of our USPs reliably dropped a
clue of a possible underlying contextual factor, such as "Boy it's been tough since
I lost my job," we had no such assurance with real patients. Sometimes patient context just isn't that important. When a patient comes in with ear pain after swim-
ming in the lake during the summer, usually it is what it is. All they will need are
some ear drops for presumed otitis externa, a painkiller, information about how
to take their medicine, and instructions on what to do if things get worse. On the
other hand, if the patient is hesitant about telling the doctor why the area around
their ear is also black and blue and acknowledges after questioning that somebody
beat them on the head, that's a different situation. The disconnect between the

patient's story and the findings on exam is the contextual red flag that something is going on in the patient's life that is relevant to their care.

The challenge we faced was how to code reliably for the presence of contextual red flags and clinicians' responses to them. We started by making a list of common situations that constitute potential contextual red flags and realized several of them are evident in the medical record. For instance, loss of control of a treatable chronic condition, such as diabetes or hypertension, is a contextual red flag. If a patient's glycated hemoglobin has gone from 7% to 9% since their last visit, indicating much higher average glucose levels, that can only mean three things: They have stopped taking their medications as directed, changed what they eat, and/or become much less active. In other words, a rising glycated hemoglobin indicates that something relevant in a patient's life may have changed, which is why it's a contextual red flag.

Other contextual red flags identifiable just from charts include patients repeatedly missing or showing up late for appointments or not following through on referrals they requested or to which they agreed. All these tendencies signify some sort of chaos or disruption that is impacting the patient's health or health care. A premise of our work is that an appropriate response to a contextual red flag is always to explore with further questioning, that is, with "contextual probing," whether there is an underlying problem that can be addressed in the care plan. Hence, if the coders agree on what constitutes a contextual red flag, then they also agree on when contextual probing is indicated.

When probing in response to a contextual red flag confirms the presence of an underlying problem that can be addressed in the care plan, as noted previously, we refer to that problem as a "contextual factor." In the case of patients with poorly controlled diabetes (the contextual red flag), asking them why they think their diabetes has gone out of control would constitute an appropriate probe. A response such as "It's been worse since I started working the night shift" would constitute a contextual factor that needs to be addressed in the care plan.

The final step in our coding schema, "contextualizing care," is determining whether the contextual factor, in fact, has been addressed in the care plan. For example, this might require restructuring the patient's insulin regimen to accommodate their new work schedule. In our coding, we have not attempted to second-guess what the best plan might be, only whether the plan demonstrates a good-faith effort to address the underlying contextual factors that account for the contextual red flag.

In sum, our assessment process, which we call "Content Coding for Contextualization of Care," or "4C" for short, is based on tracking four elements of a clinical encounter: The presence of a contextual red flag; if present, whether it is probed; if it is, whether contextual factors are revealed; and, when they are, whether they are addressed in the care plan (Figure 3.1). Setting aside the jargon, what we are attempting to describe here is the process by which one individual considers and attends to the complex circumstances and needs in the life of another. With this basic architecture in place, the next question was whether different

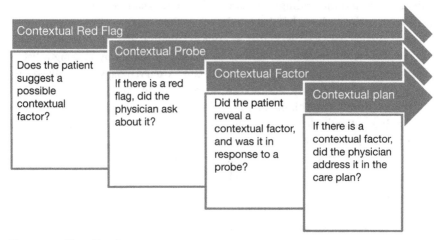

Figure 3.1 The 4C coding process.

coders would reach the same conclusions when coding the same encounter. Such "inter-rater reliability," as it is called, is a sine qua non of any coding system.

The only way to know whether there is high inter-rater reliability is to have multiple coders listen to the same audio recording after compiling data from the same medical record and seeing whether they come to the same conclusions. Specifically, how often do different coders when assessing the same interaction agree on the presence of contextual red flags, probing of those flags, contextual factors, and whether care plans are contextualized?

Initially, the inter-rater reliability was not good. For instance, two coders would listen to the reaction of a clinician to a comment by a patient that they both concluded was a red flag but would disagree about whether the clinician's response qualified as a probe. We faced many challenging coding dilemmas that our team extensively deliberated, sometimes for weeks. The result was a 54-page coding manual and subsequent training video, replete with examples and illustrations of every possible coding dilemma we encountered, how we decided to resolve those dilemmas, and our rationale.[1,2] As our four coders reached consensus on the tough calls and consistently adhered to the logic in the coding manual, inter-rater reliability reached 88% for whether a clinician had probed a contextual red flag, 94% for whether contextual factors were identified, and 85% for whether those factors were addressed in the care plan. We discuss the 4C coding system in greater detail in Chapter 4.[3]

One principle we applied across all the tough calls was that clinicians should get the benefit of the doubt. We wanted to avoid the criticism that our coding process is a game of "gotcha!" On the contrary, we wanted a system that identified contextual errors that were hard to dispute. Hence, whenever our team reports a group of clinicians are performing poorly at contextualizing care, they have reached that conclusion using a coding system that is quite forgiving.

Once we had a system in place for determining whether care is contextualized, one methodological challenge remained: measuring the impact of contextualized care on health-care outcomes. Usually, when researchers are studying how care influences patient outcomes, there is a specific outcome of interest. For instance, if a researcher wants to see whether a particular approach to counseling patients to stop smoking works, the outcome of interest is whether patients quit smoking. This is straightforward because everyone in the study is a smoker and because the outcome of interest is always the same. In contrast, there are countless reasons why patients' care needs to be contextualized, and for each there is a different desired outcome. If a patient loses control of their diabetes, we want to see their diabetes come back under control. If another patient does not have diabetes but keeps missing doctors' appointments for some other health condition, we want to see them making it to their appointments consistently. In short, the outcome of interest is complete or partial resolution of the contextual red flag, whatever it may be. This is the conceptual key to identifying and tracking health-care outcomes associated with contextualization of care. For each red flag we would track whether the red flag resolved over time.

To avoid potential bias, we assigned this duty to a member of the research team who does not have information about whether the care of any particular patient had been coded as contextualized or not. All they are provided is a list of patients and their red flags. They would know, for example, that a patient had a hemoglobin A1c of 10 at the index visit—signifying diabetes out of control but not whether the physician had subsequently identified and addressed contextual factors in the care plan. Six months later, they would look in each patient's medical record and document whether the patient's hemoglobin A1c had gone up, gone down, or stayed the same. If it stayed the same (or went up), that would constitute a "bad" outcome, whereas any reduction in the hemoglobin A1c would constitute a "good" outcome. We would then link the two sets of data together: for each encounter, whether the care had been contextualized and the patient's outcome 9 months later.

One last point: Although our aim was to assess the "impact" of contextualization of care on health-care outcomes, the study design, in fact, cannot quite do that. All we could determine is whether contextualization of care is associated with better outcomes. To prove causation, we would need to conduct an unreasonable experiment. We would have to ask doctors to randomly provide care that is appropriately or inappropriately contextualized and to verify that they had done so. If health-care outcomes correlated with contextualization of care under these conditions, we could be pretty sure the contextualization caused the difference in outcomes. Even if it were possible for doctors to change their behaviors like this, it obviously would not be ethical for actual care. Instead, we relied on observation rather than on experiment—comparing the processes in the encounters to the eventual health outcomes for red flags in those encounters.

WHAT WE FOUND

During the subsequent months, 1,799 veterans arriving at the clinic sign-in desk were told about the study by one of the clerks. Among these, 160 were not interested in meeting with a research assistant in the waiting area, and an additional 754 declined after hearing the details of the study. We told them that we wanted to learn how doctors make recommendations when a patient's life situation is a factor in their care and to see whether those doctors who had special training provided better care. Veterans learned that, to participate, they would need to carry a small, concealed audio recorder in their clothing or bag. We also asked for permission to examine their medical records. Finally, we reassured them that their doctor had volunteered to participate and that there was no risk to them for doing so.

Among those who said they would like to participate, 111 were called in to see the nurse or their doctor before we could complete the consent process and get them "wired," leaving 774 to record their visits. Even this group, however, got whittled down further. Although they all did their jobs, inevitable snafus occurred. There were 22 visits early on in which the recorders failed. These somewhat finicky devices had complex encryption software to meet VA security standards. There were another 32 instances in which the patient saw the "wrong" physician. This happened when doctors had others substitute for them, because they were either sick that day or too backed up with other patients. That left us with 720 recordings of visits with the correct physician.

As noted earlier, there was no way to know in advance whether contextual red flags would come up during an encounter. Once the visit was complete, and we got the recorder back, we would look for them in two ways: First, one of the research team members, typically Gunjan, would review the medical record going back about a year prior to the visit to see if any from a list of contextual red flags were evident in the record itself. These had to be things that a clinician should notice and that by themselves warrant probing, such as deterioration in a chronic condition, missing appointments, or not following through on referrals and tests. In our coding manual, we specified the threshold for each of these, and we set them high. In other words, the patient had to miss a lot of appointments, or their chronic condition had to get much worse, to count as something in the chart that the doctor should not miss. Again, this was to assure that we were not accused of setting unrealistic expectations. Second, if there were no red flags in the chart, another member of the team listened to the audio recording for red flags. For instance, a patient might mention that he ran out of his meds a couple of weeks ago. Or a patient might decline a recommendation such as a flu shot, which is of likely benefit. Each of these situations suggests that something is going on in a patient's life or that they have a particular perspective that is impacting their care and, hence, qualifies as a contextual red flag.

For each physician, we sought to obtain three recordings with documented contextual red flags. Because coding takes some time and we occasionally had a backlog of recordings, we sometimes collected more audio from a particular resident than we would ultimately need. As a result, in 119 instances we discarded a recording that we did not need—meaning that we had already collected three recorded patient encounters with that physician that contained documented red flags.

At the end of the data collection phase, we had a total of 601 recordings; of these, 198 contained no red flags, leaving 403 encounters in which we found at least one red flag—sometimes more. Specifically, there were a total of 548 red flags. The fact that there were only 198 recordings out of 601 that had no evidence of contextual issues that could be essential to care planning was, in and of itself, interesting to us. That was just 33%. Put another way, two-thirds of encounters contained clues that something was going on in the patient's life situation that needed to be explored because of its relevance to care planning. We did not know whether that number was high or low compared to other populations of patients. (For example, would the medical records and audio recordings of patients from a suburban upscale community be more or less likely to reveal clues of contextual issues that are impacting their health or health care?)

We then focused on what happened in response to these 548 red flags. First, we noted that physicians probed the red flags 32% of the time, less often than the 51% probing rate in our USP study (Figure 3.2). A major difference is that in the USP study we were testing clinicians with just four cases that we had contrived. In this project, we were assessing them against "whatever walked in the door."

Second, after looking at the probing rate, we determined that in 38% of the visits a contextual factor was revealed. Although many of these were revealed in response to a probe, some were just offered up by patients, which is why the contextual factor rate was higher than the probing rate. Among the 209 contextual factors, 120 were elicited by a physician probe and 89 were revealed

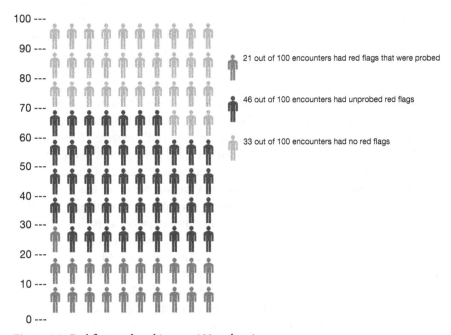

Figure 3.2 Red flags and probing per 100 real patient encounters.

spontaneously by the patient. In short, some patients fortunately will just tell their doctor what the problem is (e.g., why they keep missing appointments) even if not asked.

Third, having established the probing rate and percentage with contextual factors, we looked at what physicians did with the contextual information they had either elicited or been offered. We found that physicians addressed the contextual factor in their care plan 59% of the time and, hence, did not address it the remaining 41% of the time. This was actually better than the 22% rate for contextualizing care in the USP study. Again, it was a bit of an "apples and oranges" comparison, given that the USP study was based on just four cases. Apparently, those four cases contained contextual red flags that were, on average, easier to spot but harder to address in care planning than the ones we studied in actual practice.

We learned something else of interest here. On the one hand, factors initiated by probe were incorporated into the plan of care 68% of the time. On the other hand, those spontaneously revealed by the patient were incorporated into the plan of care only 46% of the time. Doctors need to probe more, and they also need to pay closer attention to patient-revealed factors. We have observed this result consistently across all of our projects, whether the providers were residents, attending physicians, or even health coaches providing comprehensive telephone assistance to insurance plan members.[4]

Finally, we turned to the most important question: Are we tracking something that matters? Intuitively it seems obvious that if care is adapted to patients' needs and circumstances, they should fare better. But does our coding system of contextual red flags, probes, factors, and care plans capture the benefit we hypothesize is there? For instance, if the care plan is coded as contextualized, is the patient who has been missing appointments more likely to start making their appointments rather than continuing to miss them? We decided to follow the patients for 9 months to find out.

The physicians created contextualized care plans for 123 encounters and did not incorporate context into their plans for 61 encounters. We were not able, however, to track outcomes for all of these patients. Of the 123 contextual factors for which physicians made a contextualized care plan, there were 27 instances in which no outcome data was available. This occurred if the patient never returned for a follow-up visit or the outcome of interest (i.e., the status of the contextual red flag) was never documented during the 9-month period of observation. Of the 96 remaining encounters, 68 (71%) had a good outcome, while just 28 (29%) had a poor outcome. Good outcomes were more than twice as likely as poor outcomes if the clinician had contextualized the care plan. In comparison, for the 61 encounters for which physicians did not make contextualized care plans—and for which outcome data was available—just 28 (46%) had a good outcome, while 33 (54%) had a poor outcome. Good outcomes were actually less likely than poor outcomes when the clinician did not contextualize care (Figure 3.3).

In sum, problems attributable to life context were more likely to resolve for patients whose care plans were contextualized than they were for those whose

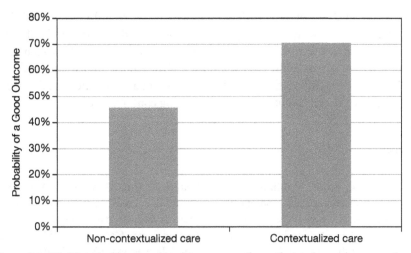

Figure 3.3 Likelihood of improved health outcomes for patients whose care was and was not contextualized by the physician.

care plans were not contextualized. In a statistical analysis the probability that this finding was due to chance was only 0.2%.

Substantial additional work would be needed to understand how this research could change how medicine can be practiced for the better. In the next chapter, we take a detailed look at how we are measuring physician performance. Subsequent chapters explore optimal strategies for using 4C to improve care.

KEY POINTS

- Patient-collected audio is a process for recording medical encounters without the physician necessarily being aware of when they are being observed. In our studies, patients record their visits on an encrypted audio-recording device. Following the visit, the audio data is uploaded to a secure server.
- Whereas USPs are an experimental method of data collection in which multiple physicians receive the same stimulus, patient-collected audio is an observational data collection method in which every encounter is different. Whereas the former is ideal for measuring clinicians' attention to patient context, the latter is necessary for ascertaining how often and to what extent that attention matters in real patient care.
- Content Coding for Contextualization of Care ("4C") was invented out of necessity when we transitioned from USPs to patient-collected audio. It was designed to standardize the process of determining, based on an audio recording and medical record review, whether each of the four steps to contextualizing a care plan have been accomplished. It also enables tracking of prospectively defined contextually relevant outcomes.

- In an analysis of 601 patient-collected audio recordings, two-thirds contained contextual red flags. Physicians probed red flags only about one-third of the time. Contextual factors were present in 38% percent of visits. Physicians addressed them 59% of the time. Contextualized care plans were significantly more likely to result in a good outcome, defined as partial or full resolution of the presenting contextual red flag.

NOTES

1. Weiner SJ, Ashley N, Binns-Calvey A, Kelly B, Sharma G, Schwartz A. Content coding for contextualization of care. Version 12.0, Released May 27, 2021. Harvard Dataverse Network Project. https://dataverse.harvard.edu/dataverse/4C.
2. Weiner SJ. Content coding for contextualization of care ("4C") (video #5 in series). https://youtu.be/ncr8azGwAqA. YouTube, n.d. Last accessed May 25, 2022.
3. Weiner SJ, Kelly B, Ashley N, et al. Content coding for contextualization of care: evaluating physician performance at patient-centered decision making. Med Decis Making. 2014;34(1):97–106.
4. Schwartz A, Weiner SJ, Binns-Calvey A, Weaver FM. Providers contextualise care more often when they discover patient context by asking: meta-analysis of three primary data sets. BMJ Qual Saf. 2016;25(3):159–163.

4

What We Hear That Physicians Don't

DOCTOR: "So you quit in 2011?"
PATIENT: "Quit smoking? It was three and a half years ago. Almost—it's
hard when your roommates smoke."
DOCTOR: "Any history of colon cancer?"

—Transcript of hidden audio recording
between a real patient and doctor

The 4C process, as detailed in the coding manual,[1] begins once an audio recording of a medical encounter has been uploaded to a secure server and the coding team has access to the patient's medical record. Audio coders are trained to systematically track and document the contextualization of care process, including when and where a clinician falters, utilizing an Excel spreadsheet or entering the data into REDCap, a secure web application for building and managing online surveys and databases. To understand the coding process, consider how the flow of a clinician–patient interaction with a contextual red flag leads to one of three possible conclusions depending on the communication behaviors of the clinician and patient and the presence or absence of a contextual factor: (a) The care plan is contextualized; (b) it's not, resulting in a contextual error; or (c) a contextualized care plan turned out not to be needed (Figure 4.1). There are two conversational paths to each.

Let's start with the shorter of the two paths to a contextualized care plan. As noted at the top of the figure, the contextual red flag could be either something in the medical record, such as a couple of missed appointments or something mentioned by the patient, such as "I haven't been very good about taking my medications lately." In response to the red flag, the clinician probes, the patient then reveals the contextual factor (e.g., a depressed mood following job loss), and the information is then addressed in a contextualized care plan (e.g., the patient

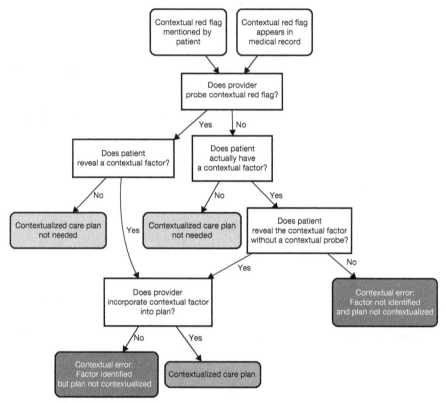

Figure 4.1 Contextualizing care: A flow diagram.

agrees to counseling). The second path to a contextualized care plan is longer and less assured: It begins with the provider failing to probe a contextual red flag in a patient who has an underlying contextual factor. Despite not being asked about the red flag, the patient reveals the contextual factor on their own (e.g., volunteering the information that they've been depressed). This time the provider is responsive and addresses the contextual factor in their care plan.

Just as there are two paths to a contextualized care plan, there are two corresponding paths to a contextual error. In the first, the provider fails to probe a contextual red flag, resulting in a contextual error due to a failure to identify a contextual factor. In the second, the provider remains unresponsive despite the patient revealing a contextual factor (with or without a contextual probe).

And, finally, there are two paths in which a contextualized care plan is not needed. In one of them, the provider probes a contextual red flag, only to discover, based on the patient's response, that there is no underlying contextual factor (e.g., finds out that the patient had missed appointments but simply rescheduled because of weather). In the other, the provider fails to probe, but it doesn't matter because, again, there was no underlying contextual factor.

Listening to a recording of an encounter, trained coders can discern among all but two of the pathways: In instances when a provider fails to probe a contextual red flag and the patient doesn't reveal a contextual factor, it is not possible

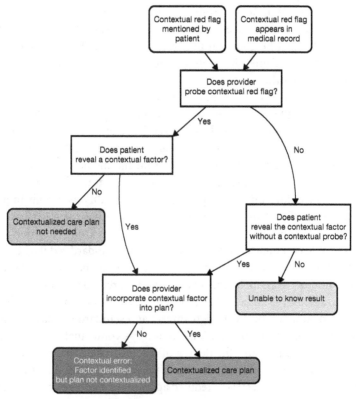

Figure 4.2 Content Coding for Contextualization of Care ("4C"): A flow diagram.

to know whether an underlying contextual factor was missed or whether there simply wasn't a contextual factor. For instance, if a patient missed a couple of appointments and the provider never asked what happened and the patient doesn't spontaneously reveal a factor, it's not possible for a coder to know whether a contextualized care plan was needed or not. Hence, in 4C coding there are four, rather than three, conclusions following analysis of a provider–patient interaction beginning with a contextual red flag: (a) The care plan is contextualized; (b) it's not, resulting in a contextual error; (c) a contextualized care plan turned out not to be needed; or (d) there was a missed opportunity to potentially identify and address a contextual factor, impact unknown. Figure 4.2 is a modified version of Figure 4.1 that takes into account these differences. In the following four sections we discuss the four steps to the 4C coding process: identifying contextual red flags (chart-based and audio), listening for contextual probes, identifying the presence of contextual factors, and deciding whether a care plan has been contextualized.

CONTEXTUAL RED FLAGS

Consider the care of a man named Don Holloway, a US navy veteran whose diabetes control recently worsened. Mr. Holloway's hemoglobin A1c, a measure of blood sugar, has gone up to 9.8 from 7.0 a few months earlier, an indicator that his blood sugar control has been disrupted in some way. The clinician's job is to figure out what might be going on in Mr. Holloway's life that could account for the change and what, if anything, could be done to help him regain control of his chronic medical condition.

Since the elevated glycated hemoglobin is a clue that Mr. Holloway may be facing some life challenges that could be complicating his ability to manage his care, it constitutes a contextual red flag. 4C coders distinguish among three types of contextual red flags: high-impact red flags, standard red flags, and audio red flags. The first two refer to data extracted from the medical record. The difference between high-impact and standard red flags is that the former are more severe. For instance, for "missing appointments" to qualify as a high-impact red flag for a chronically ill patient, we decided that the patient must have had at least 16 scheduled appointments in the medical record from the prior year and have missed at least a quarter of them. To count as a standard red flag, the patient need only have missed two or more appointments in the past 4 months. For diabetes, the cutoff between high-impact and standard red flag is a hemoglobin A1c of 9, so Mr. Holloway's value of 9.8 is severe enough to count as a high-impact red flag. The distinction between high-impact and standard red flags is useful for measuring the impact of interventions to address contextual factors. For high-impact red flags, we measure the degree of improvement. For instance, missing only four appointments out of 20 in a year is measurably better than missing eight appointments (i.e., 80% vs. 60% scheduled appointment adherence). For standard red flags, we simply look for any improvement. Any improvement is scored as a "good" outcome.

One might wonder how common it is for patients to have 16 or more appointments in a year and then miss more than a quarter of them or to take four different medications yet not refill them at least a quarter of the time—another instance of a high-impact red flag. In fact, we found that high-impact red flags are common. Some people get a lot of medical care, and many of them struggle to manage numerous medicines and complex appointment schedules.

After looking for contextual red flags in the medical record, the coder (or coding team) listens to the audio recording of the visit for audio red flags. Audio red flags are just like standard flags, except they emerge during the visit and do not appear in the medical record. In the audio of the encounter with Mr. Holloway, there were actually two audio red flags: He mentioned that he had gained a significant amount of weight since his last visit and that he had run out of a prescribed medication, an antidepressant. Upon documenting these incidentally noted red flags, the coders listened for the clinician's response to them just as they would listen to their response to chart red flags.

One of the principles for deciding whether a comment made during a visit counts as a contextual red flag is whether it has relevance to a medical problem. For instance, a comment by a patient that it has been tough since they lost their job is an audio contextual red flag if the patient is also having trouble managing a chronic condition while taking costly medications. Specifically, job loss may be part of the context for the individual's challenges in the role of patient. It is relevant "patient context." Conversely, a patient's financial troubles are not relevant if they are able to manage their care (perhaps because they remain insured). That is not to say that a physician should ignore such issues, only that for the purpose of 4C coding we only hold physicians accountable for contextual issues when there is an evident medical implication when they are not addressed. If a patient is struggling to pay for college, that is unfortunate; but we do not see helping solve that problem as a component of the physician's job as it does not generally affect their ability to manage their health.

In the absence of contextual red flags, there is nothing to probe. If our coders have not noted any red flags, we do not expect the clinician to do so either. But if we catch a contextual red flag, we look for whether the doctor has caught it as well.

As noted in Chapter 3, about two-thirds of the encounters in our study of real patients had contextual red flags, meaning that the other third of the time 4C coding indicated no need for contextualization of care. That does not mean there were not still opportunities for clinicians to improve the care these patients receive by getting to know their life challenges better. Rather, it meant that we did not identify any clear-cut issues connected to a medical problem or health-care issue that should have been explored/addressed by the provider.

CONTEXTUAL PROBES

Among those encounters with documented contextual red flags, 4C coders look for evidence that clinicians probed them. The purpose of probing a contextual red flag is to see if a contextual factor lurks behind it. A contextual factor is the potentially resolvable cause of a contextual red flag. Hence, the best probe of a contextual red flag is one that is most likely to prompt the patient to reveal an underlying contextual factor if one exists. We suggest starting with an observation ("I see your sugars are running high.") and following it with an open-ended question ("Why do you think that is?"). Our coders only require hearing the question to give credit for a probe.

Perhaps the most important principle of 4C coding is that at each step the coders formulate a model response before listening for what the clinician does. Hence, before listening for a probe, they formulate a model probe. A model probe begins with a summation of the problem ("Mr. Holloway, I notice that . . .") followed by an open-ended question, ("Why . . ."). After formulating a model probe in response to the red flag, the coder turns on the tape and listens for a substantively similar question from the physician. For instance, they might hear, "Mr. Holloway, I notice your diabetes has gotten out of control recently. What do you think is going on?" That counts. On the other hand, what they too often hear is, "Mr. Holloway, I notice your sugars have gotten really high recently. That could really harm you if you don't start taking your medications as you are supposed to." That statement does not count. It represents a failure to explore context. It is more like a scolding.

Most of the time when physicians do not get credit for a contextual probe, it is because they did not probe at all. For instance, in our example, the doctor caring for Mr. Holloway never asked him anything that would count as a contextual probe of his loss of control of his diabetes; instead, the provider referred him to an endocrinologist. The plan reflected an assumption, likely incorrect, that the high blood sugars are due to some complex biomedical issues that require special expertise.

Although sending a patient with loss of control of a chronic condition to a specialist rather than asking them what is going on is clearly a failure to probe, there were other instances in which coders heard a comment or question that seemed to fall into a gray area where it was difficult to ascertain whether the clinician was really exploring relevant context. In such cases, should the clinician get credit for probing? We developed several principles for deciding these tough calls.

First is the "awareness principle." Suppose the red flag is missed appointments and the model probe is, "Why have you been missing appointments recently?" Instead, the coders hear "Do you have any trouble getting to our clinic?" Although we consider that to be a leading question, and therefore not ideal, it nonetheless implies awareness of the contextual factor, so it counts as a contextual probe.

A second principle is to give the benefit of the doubt when it is not certain whether the provider was aware. For instance, "I haven't seen you in over a year. Are you able to come back next month?" does not clearly indicate awareness that the patient has been missing appointments—but it might, so it counts. Conversely, "I want you to come back next week to get your blood pressure rechecked with the nurse. Is that okay?" does not count. There just is no evidence that the doctor is aware the patient has been missing a lot of appointments.

A third principle is "Simon's rule," named after our late colleague Simon Auster, who cautioned us not to assume that a direct question is always the best way to get an answer. Simon's rule says that if the patient reveals a contextual factor in response to something the physician said or asked, the physician gets credit no matter what. The concept here is that a sensitive clinician intentionally may elicit information in indirect ways, based on an intuition about how to engage the patient. And, says Simon's rule, one cannot argue with success.

Consider, for instance, a physician who says "Your diabetes is out of control," after perusing a patient's log book showing a daily record of his finger stick glucose. The comment is not even close to the model probe, "Mr. Holloway, I notice your blood sugars have been getting really high recently. Why do you think this is happening?" Ordinarily, therefore, the doctor would not get credit. In fact, the comment was not even a question. However, were the patient to respond, "Yeah, doc. I ran out of insulin. That new phone refill system is really confusing," a contextual factor was nevertheless elicited. Because the physician's comment elicited the underlying contextual factor, while also demonstrating awareness of the contextual red flag, credit is given. On the other hand, if the patient had responded with, "Yeah, I know," and the doctor asked no follow-up questions, there would be no credit for a probe.

The result of these principles is a lenient approach to coding. That is, we expect to catch all the true probes and to give credit for some statements that might not intentionally have been probes. Another way to put this is to say that, if anything, the clinicians we study come out looking better at paying attention to patient life context than they probably are.

Our team met weekly while developing 4C to discuss challenging situations using these three coding principles, reviewing any discrepancy between how two different coders coded the same encounter. Often, we had what one might call "Talmudic discussions" as we parsed sentences from transcripts of audio to arrive at a consensus about how to apply the principles to ambiguous dialogue heard on audio. From these discussions, we established nine guidelines—now all in the training manual—for determining what counts as a contextual probe when there is ambiguity. Each of the guidelines is based on one or more of the three principles and designed to guide the coder in a particular situation.

One guideline, for instance, pertains to how one codes physicians' questions to patients that could represent either contextual probing or simply exploring the biomedical condition. Consider, for instance, the question "Do you check your blood pressure at home?" asked of a patient with hypertension whose blood pressure is elevated. A physician might simply be trying to find out the patient's blood pressure at home. Were the patient to reply, "Naaa, I don't bother to check my blood pressure much," a physician just looking for additional blood pressure data might reply, "Too bad. It would be helpful to know what your pressures are at home." On the other hand, the physician might be asking the question to explore the patient's level of interest in, and knowledge about, properly managing their blood pressure. If this is the motive for the question, were the patient to reply, "Naaa, I don't bother to check my blood pressure much," the physician would follow up with some version of "Why not?" It is often the follow-up question by the clinician that reveals their underlying intentions—whether simply to collect technical details related to signs and symptoms of disease or to probe for patient context. Hence, the guideline: When the intent behind a probe is ambiguous, listen for the follow-up questions and code based on those.

We stopped adding new guidelines for the same reason we stopped developing principles: We did not need any more to do the job. It is possible we will need another guideline if we come across a new situation that is not already addressed with an existing guideline. The development of our coding system has been iterative.

CONTEXTUAL FACTORS

Interestingly, although the doctor caring for Mr. Holloway never probed the high-impact red flag—his loss of control of his diabetes—they did probe one of the two audio red flags. In response to Mr. Holloway's concern about weight gain, the physician said, "Tell me about your diet and eating habits." They did not, however, follow up on a comment about running out of a medication, the antidepressant.

Once the coders determined and documented whether a doctor is probing contextual red flags in search of underlying contextual factors, the next step is to listen for whether contextual factors are, in fact, present. Most of the time this information comes from the patient's response to a contextual probe. When asked about his weight gain, Mr. Holloway described how his dentures were no longer fitting properly and how he had switched from eating fruits and vegetables to eating mostly pastas and breads, which were easier to chew. Hence, poorly fitting dentures were the factor evidently accounting for his dietary changes and resulting weight gain as well as his loss of control of his diabetes.

Not all contextual red flags have underlying contextual factors, however. For instance, had the doctor said, "Mr. Holloway, I notice your blood sugars have been getting really high recently. Why do you think this is happening?" the patient might have come back with, "I don't know, Doc. I've been really good about taking my medicine and watching my diet." Such a response would suggest that the biochemical processes in the body that cause insulin resistance may simply be getting worse over time. Patient context would seem not to be a factor.

The second way in which coders ascertain the presence of contextual factors is by listening to whether the patient volunteers contextual information. For instance, although not asked, Mr. Holloway went on to explain why he had run out of his antidepressant, noting that his psychiatrist had left the practice and he could not get an appointment with a replacement physician in time to make sure he did not run out of medication. As you may recall from the prior chapter, these "contextual reveals," as our coders sometimes call them, are quite common. As reported in Chapter 3, 89 out of 209 contextual factors, or 43%, were revealed spontaneously by the patient in our large patient-collected audio study. When contextual information is revealed unsolicited, the physician does not get credit for probing; but the contextual factor is documented so that the coding team can see whether the clinician subsequently capitalizes on the information when formulating a care plan. One striking finding that has appeared consistently in our data across several different settings is that providers are more likely to incorporate contextual factors into a care plan if they learned about them by probing rather than passively from a patient who volunteers the information.[2] This turned out not to be the case with Mr. Holloway's care, however. His physician did not address the dentures problem (which he learned about after probing) but did take care of the antidepressant problem (which he learned about despite not probing) by contacting the psychiatry clinic where Mr. Holloway receives his mental health care. This reversal of the usual pattern is likely related to lack of dental care access for veterans who do not have private coverage. (The doctor could have, however, referred Mr. Holloway to one of the free community clinics outside the Veterans Administration system, a list of which is in a handout available in exam rooms.) In most instances, however, it appears that doctors are more likely to follow through on contextual factors if they root out the problem themselves. If simply mentioned by the patient, the information often seems not to register.

CONTEXTUALIZING CARE

The coding process for ascertaining whether clinicians are addressing contextual factors in their care plan follows the same strategy as for determining whether they are probing contextual red flags: It begins with the coder formulating a model response, this time for a contextualized plan of care. For instance, given that the contextual factor behind Mr. Holloway's poorly controlled diabetes and weight gain is that ill-fitting dentures are interfering with his diet, the coder would craft a plan in which the clinician proposes some strategy for getting the dentures fixed or replaced. The coder would then give the clinician credit for any plan that addresses the patient's oral health needs.

The three principles—awareness, benefit of the doubt, and Simon's rule—also apply to coding contextualized care planning, and several of the guidelines have analogs as well. For instance, just as Simon's rule gives a clinician credit for probing even when the clinician does not directly explore the contextual red flag but nevertheless elicits a contextual factor, so, too, we give credit for contextualizing a care plan when the contextual factor is not discussed by the provider but is addressed by the care plan. Consider, as an example, a visit at which a patient volunteers, "My meds stopped coming in the mail, so I haven't been taking them." Such a comment constitutes both a contextual red flag and a contextual factor. The red flag is that the patient says they are not taking their meds. The contextual factor is the reason why, namely, that they stopped coming. Consider, now, the response: "That often happens when people don't call or come in when they run out of refills. Let's check your address in the system and then I'll put in a new order and you can pick them up at the pharmacy. Remember to call if you start running low so we know to renew your medications." We would give full credit here for contextualizing the plan of care even though the clinician did not explore either the contextual red flag or the contextual factor.

A valid criticism of this approach could be that we are not setting the bar high enough. After all, in the example above the clinician has acted on unquestioned assumptions about why the patient is not getting their medications. What if the patient's meds stopped coming for some other reason, such as someone stealing their mail? Ideally, before concluding that the patient just needs refills, the clinician would confirm whether that is, in fact, what is going on. When the medical record system is connected to the pharmacy where the patient refills their medications, such as in the Veterans Administration electronic health record, it is not hard to check. Ideally, we would like to see the clinician show more curiosity here. Figuring out why a patient's meds have stopped coming to them may involve a few follow-up questions but should not take long to sort out. Without this extra effort the care plan may simply be a solution to the wrong problem.

The reason we do not set the bar higher, however, is that our coders have no way to ask the questions the doctor never asked, and we do not want to act on assumptions either. The physician may, after all, be correct. Hence, we give credit for any care plan as long as—implicit in the care plan—there is awareness of the contextual factor. As noted earlier, the strength of this approach is that when we do report that a high percentage of clinicians are providing care that fails to address patient context and is, therefore, not competent care, it is safe to say that we are not exaggerating. If one needs a more stringent measure of skill at contextualization, we recommend unannounced standardized patients.

DOES CONTEXTUALIZING CARE MATTER?

In our study on the impact of contextualization of care, we added another element to our 4C coding: outcomes. A good outcome is defined by an improvement over time in the original red flag(s), such as a lower A1C, weight loss, or access to psychiatric medication, in Mr. Holloway's case. A poor outcome is no improvement or worsening of the red flag(s). As detailed above, for high-impact red flags we also measured incremental improvement. Missing four appointments instead of eight in a comparable time period would be considered an improvement.

Tracking outcomes is not always feasible, however. It is only possible when there is follow-up data on what happened to the original presenting contextual red flag. For instance, suppose a patient mentions that they have been unable to use their continuous positive airway pressure (CPAP) machine for obstructive sleep apnea (contextual red flag). The clinician asks why (contextual probe) and learns that the machine is broken (contextual factor). The clinician puts in an order for the patient to see a sleep specialist and have the device repaired (contextualized care) plan. Four months later, at a follow-up visit, the whole issue of the broken CPAP machine is never mentioned, and there is no record in the chart indicating whether it got repaired. In such instances, which are all too common, the coders are unable to determine whether contextualization of care was followed by the desired outcome—in this case that the patient is again using their CPAP machine.

Importantly, in order to avoid bias, we track outcomes using a blinded methodology. Hence, a coder designated to follow up on each patient several months after their visit to see what happened with the original contextual red flag will not know whether the care plan addressed the underlying contextual factors discovered during the visit. Technically, bias should not be an issue since each outcome is prospectively defined and unambiguous (e.g., glycated hemoglobin will go down or patient will report using their CPAP machine again). Regardless, blinding assures the integrity of the outcome-tracking process.

PUTTING IT ALL TOGETHER

It takes about one and a half times the length of an encounter to code the encounter using 4C. The coders employ algorithms according to the tasks outlined above while listening to the recording, pausing and rewinding as needed: formulating a model probe; documenting the actual probe heard; indicating whether it was close enough to the model to count; listening for the patient to reveal a contextual factor, whether in response to a probe or unsolicited; etc. For each encounter, the coder succinctly summarizes the findings. A coder might note the following: Patient reports weight gain (red flag); "Tell me about your diet and eating habits" (probe, awareness principle); patient reports a high-carbohydrate diet ever since their dentures got in the way of chewing (contextual factor); no further discussion (did not provide a contextualized care plan). A video illustrating the 4C process is available on YouTube, the fifth in the Contextualizing Care: Fireside Chat Series.[3]

When ensuring that coders are coding accurately, about 10% of the recordings are coded twice, with the second coding carried out by an experienced coder. When new coders join, they are checked more frequently. The purpose of the audit is to confirm that independent coders reach the same conclusions about the four data points: The presence of contextual red flags, whether they were probed, whether a contextual factor was revealed, and whether the care plan was contextualized.

In addition to providing tools to analyze the individual encounter, having four relatively precise data points for each encounter enables us to accumulate a growing database on the kinds of contextual issues patients face and how providers seek to address them when caring for a particular sociodemographic population. To facilitate population-level analysis, we assign each contextual factor to one of the 12 domains of context discussed earlier: access to care; competing responsibilities; social support; financial situation; environment; resources; skills, abilities, and knowledge; emotional state; cultural perspective/spiritual beliefs; attitude toward illness; attitude toward health-care provider and system; and health behavior. As the data grows, with hundreds of contextual factors documented and catalogued by domain, a picture emerges of the kinds of challenges a patient population in a particular practice setting faces. For the veterans seen at one of our sites, for instance, we saw that deficits in the skills and abilities domain, such as poor vision, cognitive loss from strokes, and difficulty understanding medical information, were the most common challenges. We have also identified the common red flags that mark the presence of those challenges. For other populations of patients, the key domains of context would likely differ.

USING 4C TO ANSWER TOUGH QUESTIONS

Inattention to context, and the resulting contextual error, may simply reflect the limitations that the individuals functioning as clinicians bring to the workplace. Regardless, we have no reason to believe that those limitations are irremediable. These same health-care professionals have the skill and intelligence to detect subtle physical findings or changes in laboratory values to recognize biomedical disease. They are smart. They chose a healing profession and care about patients as a group. It seems unlikely that when they overlook the comment "Boy, it's been tough since I lost my job" it is because they are either unmotivated or incapable of recognizing why such a comment may be relevant to the care of a patient who has been prescribed a medication they cannot afford. In the next chapter, we explore why clinicians with extensive education and obvious intelligence perform so poorly outside of the biomedical sphere and—most importantly—whether they can change for the better.

KEY POINTS

- 4C coding utilizes a standardized process enabling coders to assess provider–patient encounters. Coders formulate a direct and unambiguous "model probe" and a "model contextualized care plan," for each contextual red flag and factor, respectively. They then listen to what the clinician does, awarding credit if the responses are substantively comparable.
- When it is unclear whether a probe or contextualized care plan should count, 4C coders apply several principles designed to err on the side of giving clinicians credit. This avoids charges of nitpicking. As a result, clinicians rarely contest findings of a contextual error or failure to contextualize care.
- The purpose of a contextualized care plan (i.e., the desired outcome) is to resolve the presenting contextual red flag. Whether this occurs can be determined if there is follow-up data on what happened to the presenting red flag.
- 4C coding not only can determine whether a care plan was contextualized but can also pinpoint when and how a clinician failed to identify and address patient context in their care plan. As a result, it can serve as an educational and training tool in addition to measuring performance.

NOTES

1. Weiner SJ, Ashley N, Binns-Calvey A, Kelly B, Sharma G, Schwartz A. Content coding for contextualization of care. Version 12.0, Released May 27, 2021. Harvard Dataverse Network Project. https://dataverse.harvard.edu/dataverse/4C.
2. Schwartz A, Weiner SJ, Binns-Calvey A, Weaver FM. Providers contextualise care more often when they discover patient context by asking: meta-analysis of three primary data sets. BMJ Qual Saf. 2016;25(3):159–163.
3. Weiner SJ. Contextualizing care: fireside chat series. YouTube, February 6, 2022. https://youtube.com/playlist?list=PL9-b6XZZMupzmVuuwn1Ipph0dpI1fxx2d. Last accessed May 25, 2022.

PART II

Solutions

5

High versus Low Performers

"I'm the doctor, not the other way around."
—Comment by a physician who repeatedly misses patient context

Our system, "Content Coding for Contextualization of Care" (4C), is a process for determining whether a care plan at a discrete visit was contextualized. But we wanted to know more. We wanted to find out what distinguishes those clinicians who more often contextualized care from those who did so less often—even when seeing the "same" patients. What is different about a doctor who responds to the comment "Boy, it's been tough since I've lost my job" with "Sorry to hear that. It's a tough economy. Do you have any allergies?" and a doctor who responds with, "Sorry to hear that. What are some of the challenges you are facing?"

To explore the question, we went back to the audiotapes from the unannounced standardized patient (USP) study. The value of those tapes, as noted earlier, is that they enable head-to-head comparison of physicians with the same "patient." As you will recall, there were four different patient narratives, each with four variants: baseline, biomedically complex, contextually complex, or both biomedically and contextually complex. We compared five low-, five medium-, and five high-performing physicians from that study. Their performance rating was based on how well they did in each of their encounters. A physician was classified as a low performer if they never probed contextual issues in any encounter. A medium performer probed contextual issues on at least three out of the four encounters, but they neglected to create a contextualized care plan in the two variants where there were contextual factors to address, that is, in the contextually complex and the biomedically/contextually complex variants. A high performer not only probed contextual issues on at least three out of the four encounters but also formulated a contextualized care plan in at least one of the two contextual variants. In short, low performers were those who were oblivious to context, medium performers noticed and explored context but did not use what they learned, and high performers formulated contextualized care plans. The term "medium performer" is perhaps a misnomer, given that—as with the low performers—when context matters, patients of these physicians leave with the wrong care plan.

With 58 audio recordings of these physicians (two of them had only three recordings each), we asked the question, "How do these three groups of doctors differ in how they reason through clinical problems, as reflected in the ways in which they communicate with their patients and plan care?"

Asking how doctors contextualize care is quite a different question than asking whether or how frequently they do so. In contrast to a deductive approach, where we start with a supposition or theory of what is going on and then test it, inductive exploration is about starting with what we observe and formulating theories. Theories are formulated from data, ideally without presupposition. After watching a process closely and repeatedly, from various angles, at a certain point one says, "I think I know what is going on here." That is a theory. We continue to observe for a while longer, perhaps making adjustments to our theory along the way, until we realize that there is little to gain from further observation; we are acquiring no new insights, just further evidence that our theory explains what we are observing. Qualitative methodologists call this point of arrival "saturation."

Several members of our research team, together with Dr. Carol Kamin, a medical education researcher experienced in analyzing qualitative data, independently listened to the audio recordings, knowing in which group—low-, medium-, or high-performing—the clinician had been placed. Early on they listened repeatedly to a sampling of audios from each of the three groups to catalog every discernible communication behavior. The list of over 80 behaviors includes "engaging in small talk," "asking permission," "veering off topic," "addressing patient's concern," "encouraging," "using medical jargon," "typing while patient is talking," "interrupting," and "scare tactics." Once they reached saturation, they agreed they could continue to add to the list if any new behaviors were heard on subsequent tapes.

Cataloguing communication behaviors is not new. The best-known typology designed specifically for clinician–patient interaction analysis is the Roter interaction analysis system, or RIAS, named after the pioneering Professor Deborah Roter at Johns Hopkins University. RIAS is much more sophisticated than the list we developed. It has been extensively refined as a methodology for coding every utterance between a physician and patient into a mutually exclusive category. Hundreds of studies and papers utilize RIAS to parse conversations in the doctor's office so that those conversations can be analyzed to address research questions.

Our research team has substantial experience with RIAS. When we conducted the original USP study, our grant hired Dr. Roter's group to conduct an RIAS analysis of all 400 audio recordings. We were provided with a lengthy spreadsheet in which every utterance of every encounter was assigned to a particular communication behavior interaction type. We then looked to see if any of the communication behaviors were associated, either independently or clustered together, with contextualizing care or with failure to do so. The only (weak) association was with "backchanneling." Backchanneling is based on the linguistic concept that in a conversation, at any one time, one person is generating the predominant channel and the other person, through vocalizations like "uh-huh" and "sure," is sending messages as well through a backchannel. If this connection is real, it suggests that physicians who do a lot of affirming vocalizations also are more likely to contextualize care. It is an interesting association but clearly not a strategy for evaluating whether doctors are contextualizing care.

It was the absence of such a strategy, in part, that led us to develop 4C. Conceptually, the difference between RIAS and 4C is that the former codes for process and the latter for content, hence the name "Content Coding for Contextualization of Care." Consider, again, our "patient" who said, "Boy, it's been tough since I've lost my job." In the first instance—when the doctor replied "Sorry to hear that. It's a tough economy. Do you have any allergies?"—RIAS coded the first utterance as "empathic socioemotional exchange" and the second utterance about a tough economy as "legitimizing." 4C codes the exchange as a failure to probe a contextual red flag. In the second instance, the doctor asks "What are some of the challenges you are facing?" and the patient acknowledges that they are having trouble paying for their asthma medication. The doctor switches them to a lower-cost generic, noting that it works just as well. RIAS codes the doctor's question as "open-ended psychosocial questioning" and the instructions to switch medications as "task focused biomedical information giving." The utterances are then grouped into a ratio with those considered to be "patient-centered" (such as psychosocial questioning) divided by the total of all "patient-centered" and "doctor-centered" (such as biomedical questions) utterances. RIAS codes the second example as relatively less patient-centered than the first based on this ratio, and 4C codes the second example as probing context and contextualizing the care plan.

As these examples illustrate, RIAS is focused on each discrete utterance rather than the logic of the exchange. A physician is coded as more patient-centered for empathic utterances and less so for issuing directives, even when in the first instance they entirely overlook the patient's problem and in the latter plan a solution. Content coding is just what it sounds like: listening to and processing the actual content of an interaction. RIAS does not concern itself with the logic of an exchange. Each utterance is coded in isolation.

Interaction analysis is useful to the extent that the process and content of human communication are related. It is a proxy measure for what is really going on. For instance, people who ask a lot of open-ended questions in an interaction are likely learning quite a bit more than others who are doing most of the talking while in a similar role. RIAS would code a physician who is asking a lot of open-ended questions as more attentive to the patient's needs than one who is not. In most instances, that may be the case. But not always. For instance, one of our actors happened to be overweight, although his weight had no bearing on his reasons for visiting a doctor. Several doctors asked repeated questions about how he planned to shed some pounds, but none about the contextual red flags related to his inability to afford needed medications. The actor would tell them he was not interested in losing weight, but they would keep coming back to it. Based on RIAS coding, the open-ended questions would count toward patient-centeredness even

though the patient's stated preferences are ignored. Hence, without any knowledge of the content of the interaction, one can draw unreliable inferences about
whether care is, in fact, centered on the patient's needs and circumstances, or
context.

RIAS analysis does not correlate with physician attention to contextual issues
because it is based on analysis of short snippets of speech, each in isolation. As
our research team compiled their own list of communication behaviors, they were
mindful of this limitation. Clearly, identifying the differences between physicians
who think contextually and those who do not requires more than cataloging
differences in types of utterances. "Simon's rule," for instance, described in the
previous chapter, accommodates the differences in how clinicians may communicate to achieve the same end. Simon's rule gives the clinician credit for probing for
context if something they said in lieu of a question prompted the patient to reveal
a contextual factor.

Hence, our effort to create our own list of interactional behaviors and then
document the presence or absence of those behaviors was only a means to an
end, not an end in itself. The purpose was to engage the research team deeply
and rigorously with each recording in a manner that diminished preconceptions
and facilitated making comparisons. The goal was to look for broader patterns of
interaction—rather than just clusters of utterances—that differentiate physicians
across the three groups.

When one lines up our list next to Roter's, the differences are evident. Hers
is a well-organized typology designed to have universal application for coding
physician–patient interaction. Ours, in contrast, is just a long list of interactional
idiosyncrasies that we have noticed while conducting our particular analysis.
"Veering off topic," for instance, is a behavior we heard among physicians who are
most often inattentive to context. But it is not an RIAS code, probably because it
requires attention to content. One cannot know whether someone is veering off
topic unless one knows when that person is on topic.

The list of behaviors assembled by our team was compiled using software
designed specifically for content coding. Content analysis software is basically a
technological alternative to the stack of index cards once so common in college
when writing research papers. In the old way, insights and the evidence to back
them, with the source title and page numbers noted, were scribbled on cards.
The cards were then laid out on a large table and shuffled around until patterns
were noted and the thesis for a term paper hopefully, eventually, with enough hot
coffee, came into focus. Content analysis software not only reduces the surface
area needed for this work but amplifies one's capacity to identify, organize, and
analyze patterns in text or on audio.

There are several such programs, and we used one called NVivo, which calls
each behavior a "node." NVivo is designed to facilitate the approach we adopted.[1]
Once we had a nearly exhaustive list of nodes, the team members worked their
way through transcripts of all the recordings, assigning nodes along the way. They
listened to the audio in batches, grouped according to the physicians' performance, while fully aware of the performance group to which they were listening.

This "nonblinded" method is typical of qualitative analysis. First, one listens to either all of the high or all of the low performers, both to assign nodes and to discern overarching patterns of communication. Then one does the same with those in the contrasting group. One compares and contrasts until one is convinced that any distinguishing patterns one detects are really there. Finally, one listens to recordings in the middle to see if they fall along a spectrum, with characteristics of both high and low performers.

Although each member of the research team did this work independently, they conferred whenever one of them heard a new node. If one noted a communication behavior that the others had not, everyone would go back and listen again. This did not happen often because most behaviors were assigned a node in the first phase of the study. Gradually, the preliminary list became all-inclusive, in other words, fully saturated.

Over time, consensus developed around six axes that differentiate physicians who contextualize care from those who do not. Each axis runs along a continuum between opposite poles—adjectives or behaviors—that differentiates non-contextualizers from contextualizers.

SIX CHARACTERISTICS OF HIGH- VERSUS LOW-PERFORMING CLINICIANS

Flexible versus Rigid Communicators

The first axis extends between flexible and rigid approaches to communicating with patients about their health needs. Non-contextualizers are the rigid ones, controlling the pace and content of the interaction without accommodating input from the patient. At the extreme end of the spectrum, physicians are heard plowing through the visit, pushing whatever the patient says off to the side. Such encounters have a forceful, distorted quality, making them hard to follow, as illustrated here:

DOCTOR: "Have you ever had a PFT done?"
PATIENT: "No, um, I've never blown into a machine. I have a . . ."
DOCTOR (interrupting): "Albuterol, no the spirometry?"
PATIENT: "No, the . . ."
DOCTOR: (interrupting): "Spirometry, spirometry done, did you blow into a line?"
PATIENT: "No, all I have is . . . what do you call it? The peak flow meter."

Even an experienced primary care physician has trouble making sense of such a fragmented conversation. PFT refers to "pulmonary function test," which involves blowing into tubes connected to a computer that measures lung performance, a process termed "spirometry." It appears from the patient's statement, "I've never blown into a machine," that they actually understand the question.

Before the patient gets cut off, they are trying to explain that while they have not had PFTs, they do use another machine at home to check airflow, namely, a peak flow meter. The physician is too impatient to allow them to complete the sentence and incorrectly assumes the patient is about to say they have a home nebulizer, which is a machine used to blow albuterol, an asthma medication, into the lungs. The physician's interruption with, "Albuterol, no the spirometry?" seems to be shorthand for "I know you are about to tell me that you have an albuterol machine, but that's not what I'm asking. I'm asking if you have had PFTs." If the physician had not interrupted, they would have learned that the patient did understand the question—as soon becomes evident. To further complicate matters, when the patient tries again to explain that they do understand the question, beginning with "No, the," they are cut off again. Then the whole crazy interrogation begins all over again with the physician practically crying out "spirometry, spirometry . . . did you blow into a line?," to which the patient is finally able to answer, "No, all I have is . . . the peak flow meter." The telegraphic dialogue has the feel of two people who have fallen overboard and are grappling for a lifeboat. One screeches orders or questions at the other, then becomes too impatient to await the reply before starting over again. While the physician is talking, one hears the clatter of typing on a keyboard, almost as if there is a third party taking notes.

This rigid, highly directive approach is invariably accompanied by a unilateral decision-making style. The physician follows the above with, "I will give you albuterol; and we don't have Pulmicort, we have some other kind." To the uninitiated it sounds like they are saying "I will give you albuterol because we don't have Pulmicort." In fact, these are two different classes of medication often taken together. What the physician means is that they will renew the albuterol metered dose inhaler prescription (not to be confused with albuterol nebulized, which the patient does not take) and substitute some other comparable medication for the Pulmicort, which the patient is also taking. The physician then says that they are sending the patient for "blood work," without seeking their permission or providing an explanation. The possibility that the patient may not be able to afford the test or medication is never considered, despite statements the patient makes earlier in the visit about being recently unemployed.

These types of interactions are characterized by a physician having an agenda and the patient's input not deterring the physician from that agenda. The physician is the boss. They're not listening because they think they already know what needs to be done. They are oblivious to context.

Contrast such an approach with one that is more flexible and open to input from the patient. These interactions feel more relaxed. The physician's questions are most often open-ended, and they allow the patient to complete a response. The doctor pays attention to what the patient is saying, asking a lot of follow-up, clarifying questions. There is a balanced back-and-forth aspect—this is a real conversation. The sound of typing in the background is absent during conversation. The interactions usually begin with a greeting, followed by getting down to business but with the patient setting the agenda:

DOCTOR: "So, what can I do for you today?"

PATIENT: "I'm thinking of getting hip surgery. When I saw the hip doctor my blood pressure was high. I haven't seen a general doctor in a while, so I thought I'd get that checked out, but it was good today, so I had a couple of other questions."

DOCTOR: "Alright, sure."

It's not that physicians do not have an agenda during these types of interactions. You do hear them working their way through topics they want to cover. But there is a flexibility, a willingness to digress as needed before returning to their mental map. In the above example, the physician responded to the patient's concerns before more history-taking. Doctors with a flexible approach open the doors to hearing context, talking about it, and addressing what they learn in the care plan. A remarkable and counterintuitive finding, mentioned earlier, is that these visits do not take any more time. Although they are superficially more leisurely, the approach is, in fact, more focused. It is just that the focus is on the patient rather than on the physician's to-do list. Figuring out what is really going on with the patient is often an efficient means to a logical care plan because such an approach uncovers the actual underlying issues that account for the presenting problem.

Once our team came to a consensus about the characteristics of rigid versus flexible interactions, two members of the team, Amy and Gunjan, listened to all 15 physicians and assigned each physician a score from 1 to 10, with 10 signifying the most flexible. The score assigned each physician was based on listening to their four encounters (just three encounters for two physicians, as noted earlier). The concept, here, is "rigidity in interactions" and the connotative (nonliteral) meaning of it is hard to define. It is evident, however, in the high degree of concordance among the research team members listening to the audios as to where on the scale a particular physician belonged. Furthermore, the raters' scores correlated with physicians' performance at contextualizing care. The doctors who got a high score for flexibility, such as an 8, were most likely to contextualize care, while those who received a 2, for example, were among the least likely to perform well. We used the same scale for all six axes, with a high score indicating more of the trait associated with high performance at contextualizing care.

In addition to assigning scores, the investigators took notes independently, explaining why they assigned a particular score and providing examples from each audio. For instance, after listening to all encounters with a particular physician designated in our database as Dr. A., both raters assigned a score of 2 for flexibility, and one of them wrote,

This doctor generally launches right into providing education, ordering general screening and tests, never seeming to register that the patient may be there with a specific concern. He never asked questions. It seemed as though he just assumed the patient was there for general care. He never asked, "Why are you here?" or anything like that. He frequently refers to himself in the third person as in, "We as internists . . . " or "We as doctors . . ."

In several encounters, the patient had difficulty mentioning the contextual red flags because they would get interrupted, typically by Dr. A. finishing the sentence for them but not in the way the patient had intended. In other respects, the doctor seemed quite supportive. He was reassuring, encouraging, and provided a lot of instruction. Typically, when the patient brought up a contextual issue, the doctor would say "We will talk about that" but would never return to the issue.

The other rater echoed these observations. She writes that "He [Dr. A.] loves to tell patients what internists do for patients in general with such conditions," "doesn't let patients finish what they are saying," and "explains medical conditions very nicely." Overall, one has the sense of a physician who energetically pursues his role as he sees it, that is, as an authoritative lecturer who speaks for his profession to an audience of one. He will not be derailed by pesky questions or concerns patients raise about the struggles in their lives. During the encounter in which a woman comes in requesting a preoperative evaluation for hip surgery and mentions that she is caring for her ill son, he mutters, "That's something we'll have to come back to," and continues down a checklist of preoperative testing questions. He never comes back to it. The physician is "rigid" in the sense that he cannot adapt to the situation as it evolves. He is unable to bend away from his trajectory even when prompted to do so.

In contrast, the five physicians we studied who were all successful at contextualizing care were far more willing to go off track as issues arose. Consider physician Dr. L., who received scores of 8 and 9 for flexibility from the two independent raters. One rater writes, "this doctor starts by exploring the complaint—and spends time clarifying, not stopping at just one detail from the patient about her life situation . . . then, he states, 'let's take a break to go over your history' and he reviews what he's heard, saying 'you can tell where I'm going.'" The other rater, listening to the same encounter, writes, "he catches the contextual red flag the moment the patient brings it up." Listening to another audio of the same physician, in which a patient reveals that his daughter died in a domestic violence incident, the same rater notes how the doctor's openness to take it all in and respond to what he hears is a flexibility that reflects thinking contextually. She highlights a specific comment by the physician to the patient: "It's hard to ignore the fact that there's a lot of stuff that's happened to you over the last year. Do you see what I'm saying, the weight loss, your daughter obviously, the job, you know, so a lot of things have changed that might be influencing what's going on with your initial concern here with the weight loss." Other physicians, those with low scores for flexibility, ignored these facts.

Theory-Building versus Systems-Reviewing Clinicians

The second axis to emerge was a "theory-building versus systems-reviewing" approach to history-taking. "Systems" doctors seemingly structure each visit around a list of questions that they follow. The questions may be memorized or written out and kept on hand. The approach reflects a traditional method for training second-year medical school students in which trainees are taught to work their way through a standard list of questions known as the "review of systems," or ROS. The term "systems" in ROS refers to organ systems, such as the cardiovascular system or the gastroenterological (GI) system. A review of the GI system would include questions such as, "Are you having any diarrhea, constipation, heartburn, gas, etc.?" Because the questions are intended to be addressed to patients, lay terms are used (e.g., "gas" instead of "flatulence" or "heartburn" instead of "gastroesophageal reflux").

A rote, standardized approach encourages thoroughness and precision, even down to what words to use when asking questions. The ROS is just one component of the medical encounter that is taught and learned this way. Medical students are generally taught a routinized approach to the physical exam, often conducted from head to toe. Once they become more advanced, they are expected not to carry out every step every time but rather to exercise judgment about what to ask and what to examine. The point, however, is that they begin with a comprehensive foundation built on structure and habit.

Learning to do things by following a sequence also has its place in professional practice. In his book *The Checklist Manifesto: How to Get Things Right*, Atul Gawande documents how checklists can save lives both inside and outside of health care by assuring that effective processes are correctly carried out.[2] Checklists help pilots, doctors, and anyone else doing tasks with many difficult-to-remember steps that must be meticulously followed. Checklists are critical in the operating room or intensive care unit where missing a step in a series of tasks can be disastrous.

But there is an important distinction between learning a series of steps for routinizing critical practices and doing so for building a foundation of knowledge. In the former case, it is critical to follow the checklist every time; in the latter, we hope that the learners will grow beyond the foundational checklist. Each has its place. In practice, checklists keep the mind from drifting away from what needs to be done when what needs to be done is always the same. But in critical thinking, they provide a foundation upon which the mind can apply higher-order cognitive skills to address unique situations.

Exercising higher-order cognitive skills—required for critical thinking—is a key goal of medical education. In the 1950s and 1960s, educational psychologist Benjamin Bloom developed a taxonomy of learning objectives, which includes six levels of learning in the cognitive domain (Figure 5.1).[3] The lowest level, rote memorization, includes knowing terms, facts, or the sequence of a process. The second level is "comprehension," which is demonstrated by explaining what the memorized information means or what it is for. The third level is "application," which is demonstrated when the information is used as intended to accomplish something or solve a problem.

For processes that need to be done the same way repeatedly, this is as high as you go in Bloom's taxonomy. Correctly applying information to complete a task in the right sequence at the right time is the goal. But for processes that need to be individualized, that is, contextualized, three higher-order critical thinking skills

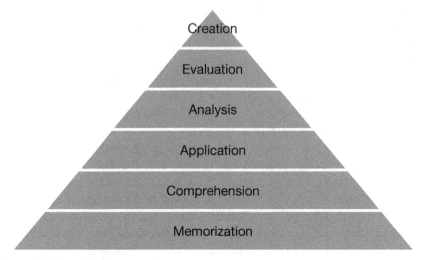

Figure 5.1 Bloom's taxonomy.

are variously required: analysis, evaluation, and synthesis—the latter also termed "creation," given that it generates a new coherent whole picture of a situation. This is what we mean by "theory-building." The requisite cognitive skills are at the top of Bloom's taxonomy. When we talk about learners lacking critical thinking capacity, we are describing the top half of Bloom's hierarchy as missing.

Critical thinking is what enables us to recognize, for instance, a discrepancy between what we are told and what we observe. A patient tells us they are doing fine, but we notice that they are losing control of their health, as reflected in rising blood sugars and blood pressure. Critical thinking also is evident when we combine data sources to arrive at new insights, as when we note that an elderly patient who has been losing weight and is scheduled for an extensive series of tests to look for a hidden cancer may have social reasons for weight loss considering evidence that they are carrying around bedding and mention sleeping in a friend's basement. As a theory emerges about the possible reasons for the weight loss, the clinician who is thinking critically will evaluate the situation by formulating appropriate questions. Higher-order thinking and the questions it generates lead to a new plan that incorporates complexity.

Exemplifying a systems-reviewing rather than a theory-building approach is physician Dr. N., who launches into a checklist of closed questions without asking a patient why they have come for an appointment. When the patient exhibits repeated confusion about medication and dosages, the physician simply keeps correcting them rather than noting the confusion as a new problem. When the patient mentions struggling to care for a parent with Alzheimer's disease, the physician ignores the comment, presumably because it is not germane to the list of questions he wants answered. This doctor is obviously also rigid, by the way.

This same physician, like others who are inattentive to data that is not a response to their prescribed questions, also seems detached from his patient as a social being. For instance, he can be heard typing throughout the interview. And when his pager beeps or vibrates, he can be heard making a phone call and conversing with a third party, all while the patient is in mid-sentence—with no apology or acknowledgment of an interruption. And when it comes time to do a rectal exam and to have an electrocardiogram—both procedures our actors were trained to decline—he just went ahead and did them without any warning, explanation, or seeking of permission. Our actors literally did not know what was about to hit them until it was too late. This same doctor also attempted humor disconnected from the patient's reality, at one point asking, "Why did you survive Vietnam?" In a population of individuals struggling with post-traumatic stress disorder and survivor's guilt, such a comment may cause incalculable harm. This provider, who received a score of 1 out of 10 for a theory-building orientation, missed all contextual red flags that were presented to him. But he got through his checklist.

At the other end of the spectrum were three clinicians who received an 8 out of 10 for their theory-building approach when new data was dangled in front of them by one of our USPs. Physician Dr. V. is the prototype, persistently following up questions and chasing leads to arrive at a new understanding of a problem. For instance, in the case of the patient who has lost control of his diabetes, the physician first asks about how the patient is taking his insulin and then keeps asking questions until the story tumbles out: The patient has trouble keeping track of his meds because of a learning disability, until recently he had help from a friend and neighbor, and he lost that support when he moved to town to help care for a parent with dementia. The clinician then arranges for the patient to meet with a nurse educator who specializes in diabetes education.

There are considerable similarities between the first two axes: The theory-building doctors are also the flexible ones, and the systems-obsessed doctors are also rigid. The terms simply reference different manifestations of their behaviors. In the former, the flexibility is demonstrated by an inclination to keep the conversation open-ended—to let it go where the patient wants it to go. The theory-building inclination is demonstrated when, following a red flag, the clinician starts to ask sequential, targeted questions that home in on the underlying issues that account for the red flag. Conversely, in the latter, rigidity is demonstrated by an inclination to herd patients through the interview, seeing the particulars of their situation, when they emerge, as a distraction from the task at hand. When these doctors adhere to a systems approach where the interview must follow the clinician's checklist, this is just one particularly scripted version of rigidity.

Open-Mindedness versus Premature Closure

The third axis could be described as extending from open-mindedness to premature closure. If a patient comes in with headaches and they have a history of getting sinus headaches during allergy season and it is allergy season, they probably have sinus headaches due to a seasonal allergic reaction. Right? But if that is the case, then why are they coming to see the doctor? Wouldn't they be the first to recognize the pattern? Hence, the red flag is that they are seeking medical care for a condition with which they are already familiar. Premature closure is a type of cognitive error that has been written about extensively in the field of medical decision-making.[4] It occurs when clinicians reach an incorrect conclusion early in the visit about what they believe is going on—typically based on pattern recognition. Premature closure can lead to an incorrect medical diagnosis when a clinician misses unusual signs or symptoms of an uncommon condition because the rest of the clinical picture points to a common condition. It leads to a contextual error when the clinician misses contextual red flags. Showing up in the doctor's office for a problem the patient is probably familiar with and knows how to handle on their own is a contextual red flag. The astute physician will ask whether anything is different that prompted the patient to seek medical attention. Hence, open-mindedness can prevent missing both biomedical (e.g., brain tumor) and contextual (e.g., domestic violence) factors that would otherwise not emerge because the clinician already has decided that they know what the problem is.

When a patient with diabetes complains of episodes of nearly passing out and says they feel better after they eat something or suck on a candy, that is a sure sign their blood sugar is getting too low (i.e., they are getting hypoglycemic). Hypoglycemia is dangerous and will prompt physicians, when they hear about it, to reduce the insulin dosage a patient is taking. In our USP case, the actor role-played a patient who was so confused about his insulin dosing because of a learning disability that he simply was not able to follow the directions without the assistance he had received from his friend and neighbor prior to a recent move. Physicians who had predetermined that they needed to adjust his insulin dosage asked a lot of closed questions, missing the larger issue and the numerous hints that there was a cognitive challenge they needed to address:

DOCTOR: "All right, so you are on Lantus [a brand name for a long-acting form of insulin]?"

PATIENT: "Lantus, yeah."

DOCTOR: "How much Lantus do you take?"

PATIENT: "Uh, I get the numbers mixed up, and that's the problem."

DOCTOR: "Lantus is a once-a-day bedtime."

PATIENT: "Are you sure?"

DOCTOR: "Right."

PATIENT: "Just once a day? Uh, that's 24 units, and um, Novo . . . Nova? Novalog [a short-acting insulin]?"

DOCTOR: "Mmm, mmm, Novolog, the super fast-acting one."

PATIENT: "Right."

DOCTOR: "And how many units of that do you take?"

PATIENT: "Uh, uh, I take 12 units of this."

DOCTOR: "Before each meal or what?"

PATIENT: "With each meal."

This exchange, and others like it, would drag on until the doctor had made a decision about what dosage adjustments to make and would tell the patient what to do. The patient's confusion was treated as a distraction because the clinician already had decided that the problem was that the patient was on too high a dose of medication, and it was just a matter of figuring out what changes were needed.

Contrast this mindset with that of clinician Dr. V., described above, who quickly elicited the narrative that the patient was unable to keep track of his medications since losing the support system that he had had in place. Interestingly, that interaction began similarly to the one above, with the physician assuming this was a simple dosage adjustment situation. However, upon hearing the comment, "I get the numbers mixed up," he switched gears to the open-ended question, "So, how are you taking your different insulins?" That inquiry changed the focus of the interview from trying to nail down what the patient had been taking to assessing the extent to which his problems were related to a deficit in skills and abilities. This led to a plan to provide special services, including pre-filled syringes, to address the patient's actual needs.

Planning Care Now versus Deferring

The fourth axis pertained to habits of deferring care planning until after further testing or consultation with specialists versus starting to plan care immediately. Physicians who performed well at contextualizing care were generally more likely to make recommendations or decisions about care plans during the visit, whereas those less attentive to context were more inclined to defer decisions to specialists or to discourage patients' questions until they could get their biomedical information needs met. In essence, they were inclined to "kick the can down the road." At the extreme end of the spectrum, a visit would consist of a triage exercise concluding with referrals to several consultants and orders to get various tests done, with no other substantive discussion. For instance, Dr. R. combined a fast-paced "checklisting" approach—"Do you drink? Do you have dark colored stools?"—with rapid-fire test ordering. When the patient tried to ask a question about what might be going on, the doctor cut them off with, "I want to do some blood work on you before we talk." She seemed emphatic and impatient with questions, frequently interrupting or finishing the patient's sentences for them. Interestingly, this same clinician also had the computer system mastered, with just brief interludes in interrogations as she paused to enter an order. Hence, it was not that she had to rush the patient along because of time lost to data entry.

In contrast to the "I want to do some blood work before we talk" orientation of physician Dr. R., Dr. P. attempted to map a plan at each visit, even before test results were in or the diagnosis was clear. Where Dr. R. would take a "let's wait and see what the tests show" approach, Dr. P. would start rendering care right away. For the diabetes patient, for instance, she attended to the confusion and struggles with self-management of a chronic condition by arranging for a diabetes nutrition educator to meet with the patient that day. During another visit, although she did not initially acknowledge a patient's comment that they were jobless, it clearly registered with her because near the end of the encounter she asked whether they could afford a particular medication. Although Dr. P. is not a "care deferrer," she is also not a "premature closer." She still orders tests, acknowledging that certain things will not be ascertainable until there is more information. But that does not stop her from exploring the relevance of patient context. Such physicians implicitly recognize that, in contrast to biomedical decision-making, which often requires ordering and waiting for test results to take action, contextual information is a continuous stream. They appreciate that each visit is a time to figure out "what is the best next thing for *this* patient at *this* time." Patients struggle with the challenges of managing their care, regardless of whether the diagnosis or the therapeutic plan has been defined.

Although Dr. P. is both attentive to context and mindful of the need for clinical information to inform biomedical decision-making, she does get distracted by the computer. This seems to be something she is aware of, given that she apologetically explains to a couple of patients that she will be typing and looking at the screen during the visit. Her ability to tame the computer-beast, however, varies. For instance, several times she concludes by summarizing something the patient had said while she was typing, but she gets it wrong. On the plus side, her summaries give the patient an opportunity to correct these errors. Regardless, despite the corrections, the typing seemed to disrupt her processing capabilities because she failed to incorporate contextual information she had elicited into the care plan. As a result, Dr. P. fell into the middle category among the three groups of physicians in terms of her 4C-rated performance at contextualizing care.

Electronic Medical Record–Skilled versus -Overwhelmed

Whereas the first four axes have to do with what one might call habits of mind— for example, whether one is rigid or flexible, goes by checklists or follows the narrative, quickly fixes on a diagnosis or remains open-minded, or prefers to wait for all the data before acting or provides care immediately—the fifth axis is more about distractibility and capacity to multitask. Specifically, it has to do with the clinician's ability (or inability, as seen with Dr. P above) to manage both the electronic medical record (EMR) and the patient at the same time. The effort of typing to document the visit while it is occurring is a cognitive drain that draws the clinician's attention away from the patient. For instance, the research team members repeatedly refer to Dr. E.'s typing as a backdrop to all of his encounters. Listening to one visit, a research assistant notes, "Lots of typing, both during breaks and while the patient is talking. . . . The doctor seems hamstrung by the electronic records." They note that the physician appears not to hear what the patient is trying to tell him. In fact, on two occasions the USP actually repeated red flags a couple of times, even though they were not supposed to do this. Presumably, they instinctively reacted to the sense that they were not being heard.

Another research assistant notes about the same physician, "Right from the beginning of appointments, there is a lot of typing, with long pauses as the physician seemed to be waiting for the computer screen."

Clinicians who invested so much attention into their interactions with the computer seemed disconnected from patients. For example, the physician might ask a question the patient had already addressed. Sometimes physicians seemed to have stopped listening or even hearing as they focused on whatever data entry task they were trying to accomplish. Instances in which a comment such as "It's been tough since I've lost my job" were followed with a checklist question such as "Do you have any allergies?" almost always occurred when physicians were distracted by the EMR. Of note, these doctors were usually systems reviewers rather than theory builders, perhaps because overattention to the computer and working one's way through checklists go hand in hand.

On the other end of the spectrum were doctors who interacted as if there were no computer in the room. Without a video recording, we can only speculate as to how these clinicians functioned so well. One approach some doctors adopt is to prepare in advance of visits, by looking over the medical records of scheduled patients at the start of the day and formatting notes in advance. This is accomplished by cutting and pasting information from previous notes that is not likely to have changed. Also, most EMRs have features that, with a few clicks of the mouse, enable providers to import the latest medication list, vitals, and previously documented medical problems into the note template. Hence, physicians who have the time and inclination can free themselves of some of the distraction of doing this work during an encounter.

Unshackled from the computer, clinicians were more likely to relax and engage. Listening to physician Dr. G., one hears occasional typing, but otherwise one would not know he is working on a computer. The clinician is quite structured, even beginning with a checklist; but the visit seems more relaxed. Although he is checklist-oriented, there is room for conversation. In addition, the clinician seems to be processing what he is hearing, noting, for instance, what he and the patient have already discussed about eating habits when he gets to the diet section of his interview with a patient who has diabetes.

Despite being a good listener and not overwhelmed by data entry, Dr. G. is strikingly lacking in conventional social courtesy. He does not introduce himself at the start of the visit or greet the patient. But he does pick up on and address transportation issues and challenges for the patient of getting to a specialist and, as a result, received a high score for contextualized care planning. Attending to the patient rather than the computer, while essential to care planning, does not ensure good "bedside manner."

Although the ability to keep the voracious demands of the computer at bay and the patient at the fore of the visit is a critical trait, and one that is associated with high performance at contextualizing care, it does not necessarily signify an affinity for building relationships with patients. Clinicians such as Dr. G. illustrate how certain traits that we tend to think will go together, such as good communication behavior and effective care delivery, do not entirely overlap. On the one hand, we have observed doctors who lack social graces but are laser-like in their focus on what the patient says and needs. On the other, we hear the schmoozers who love to talk but nonetheless miss the clues or overt concerns of patients.

Contextual versus Non-contextual Thinkers

The sixth, and final, axis is exemplified by Dr. C., who is far above average at contextualizing care while surprisingly lacking in the characteristics of high performers described above. He controls the visit, avoiding small talk and asking strings of questions interrupted by long pauses as he enters data into the medical record. His visits with patients are strikingly humorless and directive. Our team could not classify him as flexible, nor could they say that he is a theory builder. Although he is not prone to premature closure, he also is not particularly open-minded. It is true that he avoids deferring care, but this is primarily a consequence of successfully identifying contextual issues that compel action. The sixth axis includes a likely small number of clinicians who just recognize the import of context more than others for reasons we do not yet understand.

It also includes—at the other extreme—those who fail to incorporate context despite having many strengths in how they communicate with patients. Non-contextual thinkers simply do not connect the dots linking a contextual red flag to a patient's presenting problem. For instance, in the case of the patient who came to the doctor with a complaint about their worsening asthma, even while taking an expensive brand name medication, and commented that things had been tough since they lost their job, some docs just did not make a connection, despite a discussion about the contextual issue. In one case, the physician engaged the patient in a rambling conversation about how difficult the job market had become, with the patient commenting that they did not have any immediate job prospects; and the physician still did not ask about any trouble paying for Pulmicort, which cost $185 a month at the time. Without an appreciation for the relevance of context to planning care, none of the other axes matter. Interestingly, this same physician thought about the stress associated with being unemployed and commented that stress might be exacerbating the asthma through its biomedical effects on smooth muscle relaxation in the chest. But the possibility that the word "tough" in the patient's comment might mean something specific about the patient's life challenge, and its impact on their ability to care for themselves, did not seem to occur to this doctor.

The best contextual thinkers, in contrast, not only explore the implications of life challenges for care planning when they hear the red flag but then also assimilate them into all of their planning for the rest of the visit. One physician, Dr. H., after asking about the patient's ability to pay for the medication upon hearing that things have been tough since they lost their job, also considered the implications of lack of insurance later in the encounter as he weighed whether to send the patient for pulmonary function testing:

DOCTOR: "One thing I was a little bit worried, for your sake, is you know, doctors . . . we order a lot of tests."

PATIENT: "Yeah."

DOCTOR: "And I don't want to get you in a situation where you're having to, you know, choose between, uh, doing whatever it is that I come up with or I recommend and paying for it."

PATIENT: "Got you."

The physician's awkwardness is palpable as he broaches a subject that makes him uncomfortable, but one senses that mainly he is concerned about not embarrassing the patient, as well as respecting the patient's financial challenges as they plan care. At the most basic level, however, he recognizes and can generalize the implications of context in care planning.

Archetypes of High- versus Low-Performing Clinicians

Taken together, these axes illustrate the cognitive behaviors that differentiate physicians who effectively address context in care planning from those who do not and reveal that most fall somewhere along a continuum across six sets of characteristics. The archetype of a clinician who exemplifies all of the skills for attending to the complexity of context in decision-making is an individual who is flexible rather than rigid in conversation, does not let checklists get in the way of building and testing theories about what might be going on, avoids drawing conclusions prematurely in the face of conflicting evidence, looks for opportunities in every visit to provide some level of care to the patient right now, manages rather than is managed by technology, and is capable of seeing the linkages between patients' life situations and their clinical care. Conversely, the archetype of the physician who overlooks context is an individual who must drive the interview according to their assumptions about what is important, is not easily diverted from a set of routinized questions, reaches conclusions about what is going on and what needs to be done based on the information obtained from a narrow biomedical perspective, regards care planning as a last step rather than an ongoing process in patient care, is distracted and controlled by data entry, and sees patient context as a curiosity, distraction, or chance to build rapport rather than as data relevant to care planning. Using the same 1 to 10 scale employed in our analysis, Figure 5.2 shows that the highest-performing physicians are closest to the first archetype across five of the six axes (darkest line), the lowest are closest to the second archetype (light gray), and the middle performers (medium gray) fall between these two groups, overlapping with the lowest performers on EMR skill.

What would it take to move clinicians closer to the former archetype and away from the latter? Are these skills teachable? Are all clinicians capable of learning or only those who already exhibit a capacity to think contextually? Where can one intervene in the professional development of the clinician to address the problem? Should it be in practice, in residency training or medical school, or during the

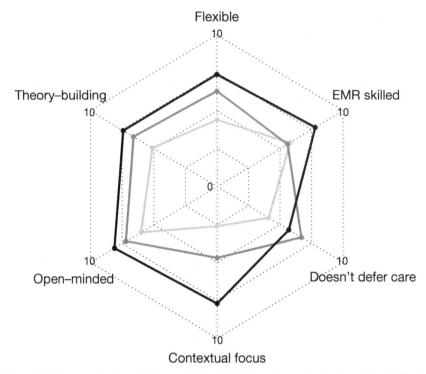

Figure 5.2 Comparing low (light gray line), middle (medium gray line), and high (black line) performers on six dimensions. EMR = electronic medical record.

admissions process? Can changes to the way we use technology make a difference? How much of the solution requires training or retraining how doctors think versus changing how quality of care is defined and measured? Finally, how might one begin to tackle these questions?

We began our examination of these questions with a narrowly constructed but rigorous study. We asked whether simply teaching clinicians—at an early formative stage in their careers—about the importance of contextualizing care, providing them with an opportunity to see how it makes a difference for the care of their own patients, and giving them a chance to practice a new set of skills would make a measurable difference. We studied this educational intervention as if we were studying a pill in a clinical trial. In the next chapter we describe this experiment.

KEY POINTS

- The audio recordings made by USPs provided an opportunity to compare the behaviors of physicians who were high- versus low-performing at contextualizing care to identify the characteristics that distinguish them.

- Six characteristics were associated with the high-performing clinicians: flexibility rather than rigidity in conversation, not letting a checklist mentality get in the way of building and testing theories about what might really be going on when a patient is struggling to manage their care, avoiding drawing conclusions prematurely in the face of conflicting evidence, looking for opportunities in every visit to be helpful even before a workup is complete, managing rather than being managed by technology, and quickly spotting linkages between patients' life situations and their clinical state.
- Physicians who performed poorly at contextualizing care tended to lack these characteristics, with a middle group in between. These findings establish a set of six axes, each a continuum, that distinguish high from low performers at contextualizing care.

NOTES

1. Bazeley P. Qualitative data analysis with NVivo (2nd ed.). Thousand Oaks, CA: Sage Publications; 2013.
2. Gawande A. The checklist manifesto: how to get things right (1st ed.). New York: Metropolitan Books; 2010.
3. Bloom BS. Taxonomy of educational objectives: the classification of educational goals (1st ed.). New York: Longmans, Green; 1956.
4. Graber ML, Franklin N, Gordon R. Diagnostic error in internal medicine. Arch Intern Med. 2005;165:1493–1499.

6

Better Teaching, Better Doctors

"I'm so glad I asked."

>   —*Medical student in workshop on contextualizing care*
>   *after hearing that her patient would have declined*
>   *a lifesaving heart valve repair because "there is no*
>   *one to hold my hand and support me after the surgery."*

We had learned that contextualizing care requires more than longer visits or empathic communication styles. In reviewing the transcripts of practicing physicians faced with our actors, we realized that contextualizing care was a set of communication, thinking, and collaborative planning skills. The physician needs to know how to ask patients the right kinds of questions, listen carefully to their responses, interpret what those responses reveal about their patient's life circumstances, and adapt care accordingly.

Based on the data we collected, it became clear that these skills are not acquired consistently by physicians during their training. Both of us are deeply involved in medical education, so we next asked why physicians are not learning them and whether we could teach medical students and residents to improve at contextualizing care.

THE MAKING OF A DOCTOR

The training of physicians in the United States is long and complex. It's hard not to be impressed by such an arduous process: the tough pre-medical courses in college, including organic chemistry and biochemistry; the subsequent breadth of basic and clinical science, typically during the first 2 years of medical school; the time in the third and fourth years acquiring clinical skills; and then the years of residency training, starting with the intensity of internship, caring for sick patients. But arduous does not necessarily mean optimal. One of us (S. J. W.)

has written a book, *On Becoming a Healer*, critiquing the process as a whole.[1] Here, we focus on one concern relevant to teaching physicians to contextualize care: Medical training tends to emphasize efficient task completion, sometimes at the expense of getting to know patients as individuals.

The efficient task completer mindset develops over a period of years through operant conditioning: In the early years of training, the rewarded task is preparation for high test performance. As a "pre-med," success is defined by consistently high scores on science exams. Successful students learn how to study efficiently, memorize by rote, take lots of practice tests, and so on. Starting with the Medical College Admissions Test, if not before, most assessments use multiple-choice questions, a format students strive to master. Unfortunately, such a format is not well suited to teaching emerging clinicians to consider patient life context. Consider, for instance, a clinical microbiology class in which students are expected to know the correct antibiotic for a particular type of infection. Whether they've acquired that skill is not hard to assess using multiple-choice questions. What gets lost, however, is assessing whether they know how to contextualize care when a patient needs more than just a doctor who knows what drug treats what bug. What if a patient can't afford the antibiotic or is fearful of taking it or lacks the dexterity or cognitive capacity to self-administer the medication? Whether a budding physician knows how to spot and respond to these situations is hard to assess on multiple-choice tests. And if it's not on the test, students are not likely to prioritize learning it.

In the third year of medical school, successful students must not only continue to perform well on multiple-choice tests but also show that they are efficient at collecting biomedical information from patients and the medical record each morning to present on rounds. These are essential skills to acquire, but they often seem like all that matters even when contextual information may be just as important to a patient's outcome. Students look bad if they don't have answers to questions about lab values, test results, or updates on clinical status, such as fevers, urine output, and so on. But they are less likely to be queried about whether their patient understands the treatment plan, has anyone at home who can help them keep track of their medications, or can make it to appointments if they will have trouble walking for some time.

By internship, the efficient task completer mindset is a basic survival skill. When one of us (S. J. W.) was an intern, before there were work duty hour restrictions, interns could not go home—even after working a 36-hour call—until every patient was "tucked in," meaning all tasks complete. Although the hours are a bit better now, the fundamental pressures are the same. A rigorous time-tracking study conducted at Johns Hopkins University Medical Center demonstrated that medical interns spend just 12% of their time examining and talking with patients—an average of 8 minutes a day with each patient.[2] The bulk of their time—64%—is spent writing notes, writing orders, and filling out forms. In such an environment, spending time at the bedside or in the exam room understanding why a patient is not adhering to a care plan or seems withdrawn or angry can feel like a distraction from the real work of getting stuff done.

With so much emphasis on prioritizing and rewarding biomedically based care for so long, how does one begin to address the deficit in preparing physicians to think contextually? This is a question we've been asking ourselves for years and, through observation and experimental interventions, trying to answer. In the following section we describe some of our early work on curriculum interventions and what we learned.

HOW TO TEACH CONTEXTUALIZATION OF CARE

When we began to think about teaching contextualization, we realized that biomedical and contextual reasoning skills are distinct. Biomedical reasoning—what medical students spend much of their time learning—involves *categorization*, or figuring out the "box" into which to fit a patient. Does this patient have diabetes? What type? What medications can be used? Contextual reasoning, on the other hand, requires *discovery*—understanding how a patient is distinct.[3] Why does this patient have trouble adhering to essential medications? What kinds of medications are available to them given what they can afford? And which are possible for them to use, given their daily routines?

We wanted our students to acquire an approach and a habit of finding out what is going on in each patient's life that is relevant to planning their care. In many ways, the discovery process we envisioned for contextualizing care is like qualitative research. Unlike quantitative methods, which seek to measure causes and effects and describe their relationships mathematically, qualitative methods seek to discover the meaning of observations without reducing them to numbers. In designing and teaching a curriculum on contextualization of care, we worked with the late Ilene Harris, professor and head of the University of Illinois at Chicago (UIC), Department of Medical Education, and an expert in both medical education and qualitative research methods.

Because contextual thinking cuts across clinical specialties and is not limited to a particular medical school course (i.e., it does not fit cleanly into the existing educational "boxes"), we looked for an opportunity for students to focus on contextual reasoning. But the curriculum is a busy one, and there is little room for adding new material. To demonstrate that learning about contextualization of care could improve student skills, we had to make the most of very limited teaching time. We also had to find the right place in the curriculum to insert the material. Our aim was to design a brief hands-on educational activity to help medical students develop knowledge and skills in contextualizing patient care at a time when they would be most receptive and available.

We concluded that the best place would be near the end of medical school, in the fourth year, both because that is where there is more flexibility in the curriculum and because it would come at a time when students no longer are preoccupied with learning the basics of how to examine a medical patient, make a diagnosis, and formulate a treatment plan. We also wanted to do the teaching in a setting where students could apply what they learned in real time to real patients. Hence, we organized a set of four weekly 1-hour sessions to occur during the required fourth-year "sub-internship" in internal medicine. Sub-interns function almost like interns (first-year residents) in that they admit and manage their own patients in the hospital but with more supervision than a full-fledged intern.

In the first two sessions of the mini-curriculum on contextualizing care, students learned about concepts and terms through discussions of cases, and in the second two sessions they applied what they learned to their actual patients. We began with an overview of medical decision-making; few medical students, or fully fledged physicians for that matter, have had an opportunity in their formal education to think about the process explicitly. (We find it surprising that the one thing that nearly all physicians do all the time—make medical decisions—is not taught. Given that one of us [A. S.] served as editor of the journal *Medical Decision Making*, this is, perhaps, a sore point.) In the 1990s, a team based mainly at McMaster University in Canada, which had pioneered the evidence-based medicine (EBM) movement, characterized good medical decision-making, which they termed "clinical expertise," as the integration of three distinct types of information. First, one needs to know about a patient's "clinical state," which refers to everything going on that is biomedical, that is, everything going on inside the body. This knowledge comes from looking over the medical record, taking a good medical history, conducting a physical exam, and ordering lab tests and other studies. The description of a patient's clinical state might include that they have diabetes and hypertension, that their diabetes is quite well controlled, but that their blood pressure remains high despite their use of an antihypertensive medication.

The second type of information is "research evidence," which refers to the best science available that is pertinent to the patient's clinical state. What do clinical trials tell us, for instance, about how best to manage someone who has high blood pressure that is not responsive to single-drug therapy and who also happens to have diabetes? There are a lot of studies on this specific question. Once one has identified the research evidence to manage a particular clinical state, in essence one has a diagnosis and treatment. At this point, it is easy to think, especially if one is a busy clinician, that one has done one's homework and that it is time to move on. Yet, at least one—and we argue two—additional piece(s) of information is still needed.

The third type of information in the EBM model is the patient's preferences. Nearly all treatments have potential side effects and risks, and information about whether those risks outweigh the potential benefits can only come from the person who will be subjected to those risks and benefits. Let us now give our hypothetical patient with hypertension and diabetes a name as they cease to be just a disease once we introduce individual preferences. We will call her Ms. Sanders. For the physician who is trying to get Ms. Sanders' blood pressure down a few notches into the normal range, choosing another medication from among a list of available options is just a moment's thought. Often, the decision is made based on the doctor's comfort level with several of the options that they have prescribed for years. For Ms. Sanders, however, the decision is about a little pill she will take at least daily, a pill that will send new chemicals to nearly every cell in her body continuously for perhaps the rest of her life. If her blood pressure is just above goal, she may prefer to forgo additional medication initially and attempt nonpharmacological strategies through dietary changes and exercise. But she may only consider that option if it is offered to her. Doctors are taught that they should pay attention to patient wishes, but few are trained to recognize that eliciting patient preferences is a systematic part of clinical decision-making.

Our work introduces a fourth type of information to the decision-making—patient context. Some might claim that it is unnecessary for the clinician to elicit patient context: One might argue that if physicians allow patients to exercise their preferences, they will intuitively take into account the contextual factors in their lives that are relevant to their care. For instance, if Ms. Sanders has inadequate health-care coverage, she would likely prefer a less expensive antihypertensive medicine over a more expensive one, if given the choice. In other instances, however, patients may not be in the best position to contextualize their own care. If Ms. Sanders were a long-haul truck driver, she might not be aware that certain blood pressure medications induce more frequent urination, particularly during the first few weeks as one's body adapts to them, and could cause significant discomfort on the road. She would have to rely on the physician to figure out what information is relevant about her life situation, or context, to choose the most appropriate medications.

Introducing patient context to medical students by showing how it is part of a larger thinking process allowed us to establish a conceptual foundation for understanding its place in the clinical encounter. "Patient context" is not just an afterthought; rather, it is one of four types of essential information integral to medical decision making and effective clinical practice (Figure 6.1).

When one of us first made this argument in a 2004 paper, Brian Haynes, a scholar at McMaster University in Canada who pioneered EBM, generously invited an editorial in the American College of Physicians' (ACP's) "ACP Journal Club" arguing for the role of context in decision-making. ACP Journal Club summarizes the best new clinically relevant research and disseminates it to every member of the ACP with occasional accompanying conceptual pieces. The article, entitled "From Research Evidence to Context: The Challenge of Individualizing Care," walks the reader through a case example of an elderly gentleman whose clinical state includes a diagnosis of atrial fibrillation, for which the research evidence shows a benefit of providing the anticoagulant warfarin because it can slightly reduce the chances of having a stroke.[4] Although the patient would prefer not to have a stroke, putting him on warfarin also increases the chances that he will have a serious bleed if he falls down. The chances of a serious fall seem to be substantial, given that he lives alone in a home where he has slipped on stairs twice. In addition, he already is taking another medication that can augment the bleeding risk of warfarin. Should this man take warfarin?

We began the first of the four sessions with one of several cases similar to these examples that illustrate how arriving at an appropriate care plan requires consideration of context. We found it particularly effective to begin by presenting only information about the clinical state and asking students what they would do.

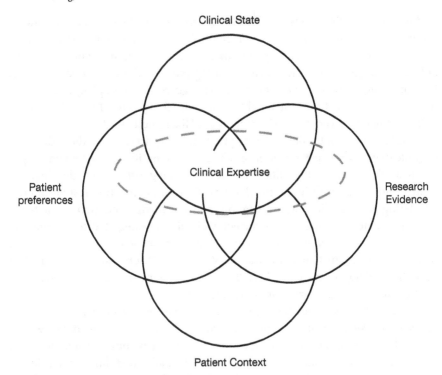

Clinical State

Patient
preferences

Clinical Expertise

Research
Evidence

Patient Context

Figure 6.1 Adding context to a model of clinical expertise. Modified from Haynes RB, Devereaux PJ, Guyatt GH. Clinical expertise in the era of evidence-based medicine and patient choice. BMJ Evidence-Based Medicine 2002;7:36–38.

Most of them had diligently learned the relevant research evidence, so they were eager to respond. Then, we would throw in a twist by asking them about patient preferences and revealing what the patient said they wanted. Our students would discover that patients do not necessarily prefer what they had assumed patients would prefer. Not everyone thinks, for example, that a 2% annual reduction in risk of a stroke—a typical average benefit of taking warfarin (which was the only option at the time)—is worth the hassle of continuous monitoring with blood testing and the risk that if they fall down or end up in a car accident they are at increased risk of severe bleeding. Finally, once the students had thought about all that, we would throw in contextual factors—competing responsibilities, financial challenges, the loss of social support, etc.—and ask them what they would do. Our goal was to walk novice clinicians through a process that illustrates how skipping steps, particularly the steps that they have not been sensitized to think about systematically, can result in an inappropriate and even dangerous plan of care.

Hence, our mini-curriculum was designed to provide a foundation for incorporating contextual thinking into medical decision-making. Over the course of the first two sessions, we also introduced the 10 domains of patient context (later expanded to 12) and provided examples to illustrate how each domain could alter what makes sense in the care of a particular patient. We drew analogies from traditional biomedical decision-making concepts. For instance, medical students routinely are taught to formulate a *differential diagnosis* for their patients—a list of possible causes of a patient's symptoms in order of likelihood—and to use their differential diagnosis to guide their reasoning process. The differential diagnosis for worsening asthma includes new allergic triggers, gastroesophageal reflux disease, and viral infections. We taught them to develop a *contextual differential* as well, in which they were to consider, in order of likelihood, the domains of context that could contribute to their patient's problems. They were to use those domains to guide their contextual reasoning and help them identify which domains might be involved. The contextual differential for worsening asthma includes financial factors impacting on ability to purchase medications, competing responsibilities interfering with medical administration, and knowledge and skills deficits regarding how to take medication correctly. Finally, we integrated these concepts and terms into the series of steps that would later become our coding system, "Content Coding for Contextualization of Care" (4C). Our students learned to be on the lookout for contextual red flags, to probe for contextual factors, and to incorporate what they learned into the care plan.

The second two sessions took students, and what they had learned, literally to the bedside. We began in the conference rooms, located on the medicine wards, where they were accustomed to meeting. Instead of pulling out another case, we would ask them to talk about patients they had admitted during the prior 24 hours. For each, we would challenge them to identify a contextual red flag. Some of the stories told in earlier chapters came from these sessions. For instance, the opening account in Chapter 1 of Amelia Garcia originated from a student presentation and follow-up bedside visit. As described, Ms. Garcia had been admitted the previous night for hemodialysis with her usual fluid overload and electrolyte abnormalities. She would have gone home that afternoon with no follow-up plan other than the usual admonishment not to miss her hemodialysis again in the future. However, a student participating in our educational intervention recognized, following a discussion of the case, that this patient's recurring emergency room visits for a preventable problem constituted a contextual red flag. With some new conceptual tools in hand, she made her way with our team in tow to the patient's room, where she interviewed Ms. Garcia with help from a bilingual classmate.

The educational value of these bedside learning experiences—apart from their potential quality-of-care benefit for patients—was that they were an epiphany for students. The students had seen the patient admitted and analyzed and assessed by multiple physicians and other staff to arrive at what seemed to be an appropriate care plan. To then discover that relevant issues had been overlooked and that the care plan was inappropriate—that turned on a light bulb.

The extent to which these "aha" moments appeared to have the desired effect varied considerably from student to student. By their fourth year, medical students have been indoctrinated to varying degrees into a narrow biomedical model. Although for one student the discovery that Ms. Garcia had been repeatedly admitted and put at unnecessary risk because nobody thought to find out that she needed to have her dialysis moved to a more convenient location was a big deal, for another student it just was not of interest. In fact, some students were offended and found it inappropriate that we were returning to patients' bedsides to ask them questions when we were not a part of the care team, even when the attending in charge of the patient and the patient had given consent. It was as if all the attention to patients' psychosocial situations, and the intimate questions such attention entailed, seemed somehow off to some students. Reactions sometimes bordered on hostile.

When we asked students why they thought they and their teams tended not to explore patient context, we got essentially four answers. The first was that they do not like asking questions when they think they will not know what to do with the answers. The second was that once we ask patients about their life situations, it might open a Pandora's box; and there are too many other things to deal with already. The third answer we received was that asking patients about their life situations could trigger emotional outpourings, and the students feared they would not be comfortable with that. And fourth, some said that they just did not think it was their job.

Medical training reinforces the notion that learning and practicing medicine are about applying knowledge from fields such as biochemistry, physiology, and pathology and, of course, clinical research, to prescribe treatments or preventions for various conditions. There is also a variable amount of didactic pre-clinical teaching about the biopsychosocial model of care, but it rarely gets mentioned in the clinical setting. Our hope was that this brief educational intervention would serve as a jolt against the prevailing current. We were interested to see whether it was having any effect.

TESTING THE TEACHING

Teaching contextualization of care successfully would mean that the students become skilled at probing contextual red flags and incorporating contextual factors in care planning. We wanted to show convincingly that these were learnable skills and that even our brief workshop could improve them measurably.

A simple approach would be to teach some students these skills and then test them using standardized patients. At UIC, as at most medical schools, and as part of the required national US Medical Licensing Examination (USMLE) Step 2 exam at the time, our students were assessed for a variety of skills with standardized patients, so they were accustomed to the experience. Furthermore, because we still were working with the actors from our unannounced standardized patient (USP) study, we could ask the same actors to portray the same cases that we had used in the USP study—cases we already knew posed challenges for practicing physicians.

We set out to conduct a randomized controlled educational trial. Carrying out such a study is not easy or cheap. One reason there are so many fewer educational than clinical trials is that there are fewer sources of funding for educational research. However, the National Board of Medical Examiners (NBME)—the developers of the USMLE tests—annually awards one or two Edward J. Stemmler, MD, Medical Education Research Fund grants. These grants reflect NBME's commitment to studying and improving methods for assessing medical skills. We were fortunate to obtain a Stemmler grant, which enabled us to conduct our study using the fourth-year medical student class at UIC.

For 15 months, during month-long internal medicine sub-internships at two neighboring hospitals, we taught the contextualization workshop at one hospital and not at the other. We alternated hospitals for the workshop to separate the effect of the workshop from the effect of the clinical site. Medical students at UIC are assigned to their sub-internship months and hospitals based on a random lottery process, with six to eight students per hospital per month. By repeating the workshop with half the students each month, we made sure that both groups had students earlier and later in their medical training.

At the end of each month, both groups of students came to our clinical performance center and interviewed four standardized patients—the same four cases and actors that we had used in the USP study described earlier. And, as in the USP study, we measured whether students noticed and probed both biomedical and contextual red flags and whether they incorporated unusual biomedical and contextual factors, when present, into their care plans. We took special care to be sure that the people who were listening to recordings of the interviews or reviewing the students' care plans were blinded, meaning they had no knowledge of whether the student had been in a workshop group or not.

We expected that students who had been in the workshop would be better than those who had not been at probing contextual red flags and at contextualizing their care plans when they discovered a contextual factor. We also anticipated that we would not see any difference in probing biomedical red flags or incorporating biomedical factors into care plans, although we wanted to be sure in case attention to patient context turned out to be a distraction from biomedical reasoning.

Our results were affirming. We had 124 students participate in the study and the standardized patient assessments. Students who had taken the workshop probed contextual red flags 86% of the time, while those who had not only probed them 61% of the time. For biomedical red flags, however, both groups probed them 77% of the time. Similarly, students who had taken the workshop contextualized their care plans in 67% of the encounters with a contextual factor, while those who had not taken the workshop only contextualized in 24% of these encounters. Again, there was no difference among the two groups in adapting care plans to biomedical factors. Further analysis showed that although probing for context made contextual planning more likely, the workshop group was better at planning than the other students, even in cases in which both groups probed. We published these results in *JAMA: The Journal of the American Medical Association*, and the journal featured our study in its JAMA Report video series.[5]

We were happy to find that medical students could demonstrate improvement after even such a brief intervention. We then introduced the same workshop and conducted a second randomized trial with resident physicians and standardized patient assessments. This follow-up study was part of the research described in Chapter 3 that additionally employed real patient-collected audio assessments. Once again, as measured with standardized patients, residents who had received our 4-hour workshop were more likely to contextualize their care plan (65% for workshop participants vs. 43% for others). Unfortunately, however—as we describe below—some important limitations to our educational intervention emerged when we tested the residents' performance with real patients.

THE GAP BETWEEN COMPETENCE AND PERFORMANCE

We had demonstrated that we could teach medical students and residents enough about contextualization of care that they could demonstrate improved skills when tested. That is, we had improved the competence of our learners. Competence is necessary for successful performance: If one does not know how to do something correctly, one will not reliably do it correctly. But competence is not the same as performance. We can know how to draw a bow and hit a target alone at an indoor archery range, but doing the same in an outdoor archery competition in the face of wind and other competitors may be substantially more difficult.

Our workshop study with the medical students led to a surprising discovery in this vein. We had used the same cases and actors to test our students as we had in the USP study with practicing physicians. Table 6.1 compares the success of our trained students, our untrained students, and the practicing physicians.

Not only did our trained students do better at contextual probing and care planning than the practicing physicians, our untrained students were better as well. But that is not because medical students are better than attending physicians—it is because the medical students who succeed are demonstrating competence in a controlled situation when they know they are being tested, while the practicing physicians who succeed are demonstrating real-world performance when they do not know they are being tested. That is a higher standard and a harder test.

In 1990, George Miller, one of the founding figures in the study of medical education, proposed a four-level hierarchy of assessment, popularly called "Miller's

Table 6.1 Comparison of Probing and Planning Rates Among Students (with Standardized Patients) and Practicing Physicians (with Unannounced Standardized Patients)

	Trained Students/ Tested in Lab	Untrained Students/ Tested in Lab	Practicing Physicians/USPs in Their Offices
Biomedical probing	77%	77%	65%
Contextual probing	86%	61%	46%
Correct care plan when there was a contextual factor present	67%	24%	21%

Pyramid." The hierarchy is "knows," "knows how," "shows how," and "does." Each succeeding level is more important and more difficult to assess. We had proven that our workshop improved contextualization at the "shows how" level; learners could demonstrate contextual care with standardized patients. But we also knew that seeing an effect on performance outside of testing conditions—the "does" level—would be much more meaningful. Did the residents who had our workshop contextualize care with their real patients more often compared with the residents who had not had the workshop?

Unfortunately, no. In the audiotapes where our team heard contextual red flags, residents probed those flags 27% of the time, regardless of whether they had been through our workshop or not. When our team heard contextual factors that should have been incorporated into care plans, residents incorporated those factors 34% of the time, also regardless of whether they had participated in the workshop or not. And, as a result, the health outcomes of the patients, which were more likely to improve when their doctors contextualized care plans, were no different in the two groups.[6]

Thus, one of the lessons of our studies is that although one can improve skills with a mini-course, without a more impactful intervention one apparently cannot in 4 hours of training transform how physicians approach their daily work. What kind of intervention, then, is required for real change (i.e., to alter clinician performance)? Looking for answers, we came upon literature describing the method of "audit and feedback," an effective strategy in studies of other interventions designed to change physician practice.[7] In brief, altering something as complex as how doctors take care of patients often requires frequent reinforcement. Technology can also be an important aid.[8] We planned our next moves.

KEY POINTS

- Medical training and the practice environment reinforce an "efficient task completer" mindset and appear to devalue attention to individual patient characteristics that are essential to planning effective care.
- Brief intensive educational interventions that combine both didactic and experiential learning can be effective at teaching demonstrable skills at contextualizing care, when assessed in a standardized patient laboratory.
- These newly acquired skills, however, are not carried over into actual practice. This "skills-to-performance gap" reflects the difference between how learners perform when they know they are being tested and what they do in actual practice.
- Hence, while medical education interventions will likely play an important role in teaching essential skills at contextualizing care, they are not likely sufficient to change how clinicians practice. Changing practice may require an ongoing process of continued assessment and reinforcement in the practice setting.

NOTES

1. Weiner SJ. On becoming a healer: the journey from patient care to caring about your patients. Baltimore: Johns Hopkins University Press; 2020.
2. Block L, Habicht R, Wu AW, et al. In the wake of the 2003 and 2011 duty hours regulations, how do internal medicine interns spend their time? J Gen Intern Med. 2013;28(8):1042–1047.
3. Weiner SJ. Contextualizing medical decisions to individualize care: lessons from the qualitative sciences. J Gen Intern Med. 2004;19(3):281–285.
4. Weiner SJ. From research evidence to context: the challenge of individualizing care. ACP J Club. 2004;141(3):A11–A12.
5. Schwartz A, Weiner SJ, Harris IB, Binns-Calvey A. An educational intervention for contextualizing patient care and medical students' abilities to probe for contextual issues in simulated patients. JAMA. 2010;304(11):1191–1197.
6. Weiner SJ, Schwartz A, Sharma G, et al. Patient-centered decision making and health care outcomes: an observational study. Ann Intern Med. 2013;158(8):573–579.
7. Ivers N, Jamtvedt G, Flottorp S, et al. Audit and feedback: effects on professional practice and healthcare outcomes. Cochrane Database Syst Rev. 2012;(6):CD000259. DOI: 10.1002/14651858.CD000259.pub3.
8. Sutton RT, Pincock D, Baumgart DC, Sadowski DC, Fedorak RN, Kroeker KI. An overview of clinical decision support systems: benefits, risks, and strategies for success. NPJ Digit Med. 2020;3:17.

7

Is Lasting Change Possible?

"Wow, my grandmother could do better than this. She has common sense."
—*Comment by an attending physician after reviewing*
a report based on audio recordings of physician
interactions with patients in her clinic

Regardless of how much education clinicians have had about contextualizing care, once in the exam room—typically seated in front of a computer with a patient sitting nearby—they are pulled in other directions. First, there's the list of tasks they need to accomplish: If a patient is there for a primary care visit, there are screening tests to discuss, patient concerns to address, labs and procedures or consultations to order, and medications to renew. In such a setting it's easy not to ask a patient who isn't using their continuous positive airway pressure (CPAP) machine, for instance, why. After all, patients are often "non-compliant" with CPAP. Several times we've collected audio recordings of visits in which a physician either ignored evidence a patient wasn't using their CPAP or simply told them it was important to use it without asking why they weren't. Contrast that with one recording in which the physician did ask and the patient replied, "I got a lot going on in my life." The provider continued with "Can you tell me more?" The patient responded that he was under a lot of financial stress and was also in the process of moving and starting a new relationship. He said he felt overwhelmed and distracted and mentioned that he was uncomfortable with how the CPAP machine could affect sex and physical intimacy. The doctor asked the patient if he thought it would be helpful to see a mental health counselor and, perhaps, a social worker. The patient agreed that he might benefit from both. This clinician had picked up on two domains of patient context—emotional state and financial situation—based on a single red flag (i.e., that the patient had stopped using his CPAP). This example begs the question, "How do we get more physicians to adopt such an approach?"

In the prior chapter we learned that it's not sufficient simply to train physicians to contextualize care. As we saw, acquiring the skill was insufficient to change how they practice. Medical education is a vital first step but apparently not sufficient. There are too many other priorities and pressures in actual practice. Several stand out. First, physicians are tracked by a wide range of other performance measures, motivating them to order screening tests, offer vaccinations, prescribe various medications based on guideline recommendations, and so forth. There is no measure of contextualization of care. Second, given the time constraints of the visit, physicians fear getting mired down in what may seem like intractable problems in their patients' lives, skeptical that anything they do will make a difference. And third, they spend much more time staring at a screen than getting to know their patient. Medical record systems prompt physicians to order screening tests, avoid drug interactions, select billing codes, write highly structured notes, and so forth. They do not prompt them to ask their patient why they haven't been using their CPAP machine.

With these factors in mind, we've designed and tested quality improvement (QI) interventions to facilitate attention to patient life context in care planning. In this chapter we describe three of them. The first two employ audit and feedback, one using patient-collected audio and the other unannounced standardized patients (USPs). For years we'd used these methods to audio-record clinical interactions for research purposes, to study contextualization of care. A natural next step was to share the data and our analysis with the providers themselves, in the hope that it would enable them to see where they are performing well and where they might want to improve. The third intervention consists of building clinical decision support (CDS) tools into the electronic health record system, tools that guide clinicians to contextualize care. In contrast to current CDS, which draws on guidelines and algorithms intended to standardize care, the CDS innovations we pursued were designed to help clinicians customize—or, as we say, contextualize—care.

PATIENT-COLLECTED AUDIO FOR AUDIT AND FEEDBACK

In order to harness 4C as a QI strategy we had to transition from conducting research to applying what we'd learned in practice. In the health-care field this is often referred to as "translation." Translation means taking something that has been shown effective in basic or clinical studies and introducing it into the actual practice setting so that people can benefit from what has been learned. We had documented, through our research, that 4C measures contextualization of care and that contextualization of care predicts patients' health-care outcomes. Now we wanted to use 4C as a performance measure to drive improvement in contextualization of care by showing the data to clinicians—both what they are doing well and where they are missing opportunities to contextualize care. How to proceed?

The most significant difference between carrying out this work as QI and as research is that providers cannot opt out of QI. Participating in QI is not generally optional. A clinician would not get far saying to management, "You know, I'm just not comfortable having you monitor whether my patients are getting colonoscopies, so I'd prefer if you left me out when you collect that data." Allowing providers to opt out, particularly those with low performance, undermines the mission.

In contrast to research, which is monitored by an institutional review board, QI is monitored by a QI committee. Another difference is that QI is intended to have a lasting effect on patient care. It is possible that knowing that an intervention is QI and not research may itself be motivating. If providers have the impression that all this audio recording is just part of some study that will be over soon, it is easy to assume an attitude of "this too shall pass." On the other hand, if they understand that there is no plan to discontinue providing the feedback, they can see that contextualizing care is truly valued at their organization. Hence, we referred to our proposed intervention as a QI "program" rather than as just a "project."

Getting Buy-In

Although physicians are accustomed to being assessed across a range of quality indicators, there is a difference between having one's orders or notes audited and being audio-recorded while caring for patients. Early on, we formulated three basic principles to anticipate and address participant concerns. Each applies to physicians and patients alike. The first is that the program must feel safe. Providers will embrace feedback only if confident that the data does not identify them and could not get them in trouble with management. For patients, we found that the major concern is the potential that it might put their doctors at risk. In addition, patients need to be sure that their confidentiality is protected as well. We explained to both parties that the data is stored at the same level of security as a patient's medical record and that all identifiers—patients' and physicians'—are removed before findings are shared (except when physicians request to see their own data).

The second principle is to implement the audio-recording program in such a way that it is not an additional work burden for participants. Patients should never be delayed in seeing their doctors because we are holding them up explaining the project in the waiting area. We also agreed to avoid disrupting physicians' workflow. We sought ways to embed the feedback into physicians' regular standing meetings.

The third principle is that the value of the project should be evident to both doctors and their patients. We discovered early on that the most compelling findings are the real-life examples we compile rather than the quantitative data. Each case that we share to illustrate high or low performance is organized according to the 4C framework: First, there is a red flag, then a probe or the absence thereof, then a contextual factor revealed, and then a care plan that is either contextualized or not. A report handed to a small group of physicians with 5–10 such examples—with their knowledge that all these patients were seen by one of them in the previous month—has unmistakable relevance, particularly when the errors are consequential. For instance, when shown something they overlooked that prevented a patient from following a treatment plan that they themselves had recommended, it is hard for them to conclude that "this doesn't seem useful." In addition to the value of such feedback, we've arranged for participating physicians to get 20 hours per year of credit toward their board recertification requirements (called "Maintenance of Certification," or MOC), which they appreciate.

Convincing patients of the value of the project seems to depend on their perceptions of the care they receive. When our team recruits veterans, they sometimes respond, "You don't need to look at my doctor here in the general medicine. You should be taping those guys upstairs in the specialty clinics" or "You ought to record those clerks over there . . . the way they treat people!" We emphasize that we are just as interested in collecting data on excellent care as on care with problems. Finally, we've seen how veterans care about each other. We hear comments like, "Well, if this will help a brother, I'm all for it."

Getting Authorization

With these principles as a guide, beginning in 2012, we initiated a process of implementing the program at two sites–Jesse Brown Veterans Affairs (VA) Medical Center and Edward Hines, Jr. VA Hospital—where we had conducted much of our prior research. We already had the long-standing support of Veterans Integrated Services Network 12 (VISN 12) director Jeffrey Murawsky, who had assisted us during the research phase when he'd been the VISN chief medical officer, as described in Chapter 2. Jeff agreed to allocate VISN funds—what amounted to about $130k per year, to cover the costs of the program.

Before getting started, however, we had work to do: First, we reviewed the audio-recording protocol with the attorney designated to provide legal counsel at these facilities. She confirmed that the process was lawful as long as veterans volunteered without coercion to carry an audio recorder and employees were informed that they could be recorded. We also conferred with the facilities' privacy officers, who are responsible for certifying that both clinical and research protocols meet privacy standards for protecting patients' sensitive data. After demonstrating our encryption practices and indicating the server space we use, the project was approved.

Our next visit was to the medical centers' union stewards to seek their support. The unions are not authorized to interfere with patient care processes, including QI, as long as the processes do not impact working conditions, such as job duties or employee compensation. We were well advised, however, that it would be prudent for the union stewards to hear about our project from us first because a protocol involving concealed audio recording of employees could spark paranoia that could undermine the goals of the initiative.

The process for communicating with the union stewards was somewhat different at the two facilities. At Jesse Brown, Saul met with each of them one-on-one, after reaching out by email. Afterward, he presented the protocol to the hospital's quality committee, which approved it. At Hines Hospital, however, union stewards are invited to attend the quality committee meetings to learn about new initiatives, and they also receive the minutes. When Saul was presented to the Hines committee, a union steward who was there raised no concerns. The program was approved. Two years later, despite no complaints from participating providers, a new union president objected vociferously to the program. She raised spurious concerns, including that we were spying on patients for the government and that we did not have appropriate approvals. She also had strong political clout related to connections to a federal official seeking re-election. The VA can become a political football at times, and sometimes programs and individuals are affected. The program was suspended at Hines pending a formal investigation, which found no evidence to support her concerns, and then subsequently resumed.

When we introduced the project to the physicians, we emphasized that the data was for them alone. We said, "This is solely for your professional development and to benefit your patients." The unstated but implied message was that "If you choose to disregard what we share with you, your patients will continue to get suboptimal care, and you will continue to see reports—whether you look at them closely or not—that show the same problems without improvement." As one attending physician put it at one of the meetings where we shared the findings, "Wow, my grandmother could do better than this. She has common sense." That was the kind of response for which we hoped.

Getting Started

Data collection began uneventfully, with staff setting up tables in or near waiting rooms with posters advertising the program. They handed out flyers in the waiting area to patients who were waiting for their appointments. Veterans varied substantially in their reactions to the opportunity. We trained the staff to discourage participation whenever a veteran seemed reluctant. Close to 40% of those who expressed interest took a recorder into their encounter. Nevertheless, physicians sometimes told us that veterans—who had seemed enthusiastic about participating in the waiting room—would tell them that they had been recruited to spy. We redoubled our efforts to message clearly that the program is entirely voluntary, that clinicians support it, and that the findings are used exclusively to help them improve their care.

Our first indication that the program had a lot to offer came when we presented the first round of data to physicians and other members of the health-care team at an all-staff meeting at Jesse Brown in March 2013. We documented that physicians were probing only about 40% of the contextual red flags and incorporating just 45% of identified contextual factors into care plans. In other words, we saw evidence that these issues were attended to in less than half of all cases where there were contextual issues relevant to care planning. This would serve as a baseline upon which to improve. Each subsequent report would show a graph, as in Figure 7.1, of both the probing and contextualized plan of care (POC) rate over time, with a summary along the bottom axis of the numbers of physicians participating in various meetings and other activities we arranged to improve their performance. Originally, we shared the data using handouts but eventually changed over to slide decks.

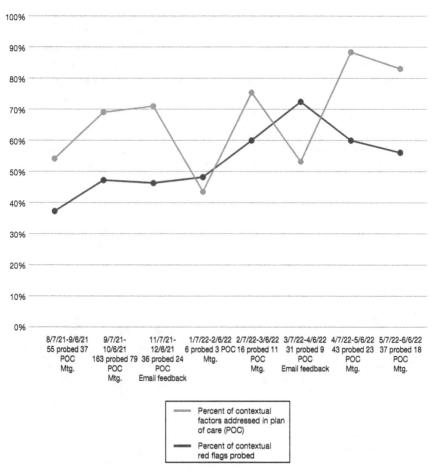

Figure 7.1 Changes with feedback in the percentage of contextual red flags that are probed ("Probe") and the percentage of contextual factors addressed in plans of care ("POC") at one clinic. Educational interventions and participation levels noted. Mtg. = meeting. Reprinted with permission from Weiner SJ, Schwartz A, Sharma G, et al. Patient-collected audio for performance assessment of the clinical encounter. Jt Comm J Qual Patient Saf. 2015;41(6):273–278.

The Program Evolves

We subsequently added several charts and graphs to provide a visual under-standing of data that we thought would be useful. They include the following:

- A two-shaded pie chart titled "How the red flag presented?": It shows the proportion of red flags found by our coders in the medical record and the proportion heard while listening to an audio recording of the visit. This is useful in illustrating how important it is not to rely only on the medical record or only on the patient interaction to identify indicators that a patient is struggling with life issues that may be directly relevant to planning their care (Figure 7.2, left side).
- A bar graph titled "Types of red flags": It shows how red flags sort into a typology our team developed through a qualitative analysis of nearly 3,000 4C-coded encounters.[1] The findings provide useful data to clinicians about what to look out for in different practice settings. For instance, in one clinic, uncontrolled chronic conditions might account for a plurality of contextual red flags. In another, it could be medical equipment and supplies adherence (Figure 7.3).
- A two-shaded pie chart titled "Percentage of red flags probed" showing cumulative performance since the start of data collection at a site (in contrast to the run chart in Figure 7.1, which shows change over time).

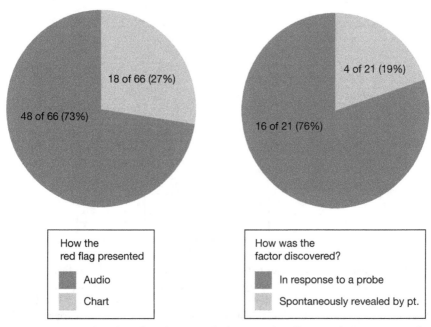

Figure 7.2 Examples of 4C data sharing with clinicians that illustrate the importance of looking and listening for red flags and probing them to elicit patient context.

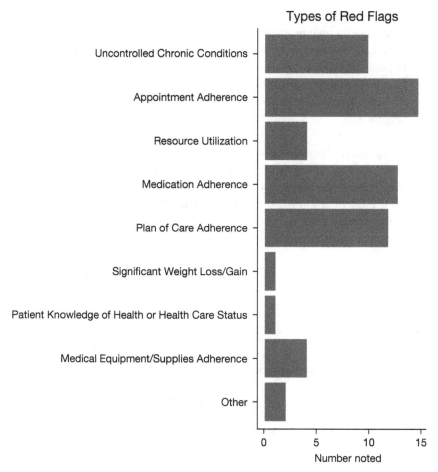

Figure 7.3 Example of 4C data sharing with clinicians about the types and relative frequencies of red flags among patients seen at their clinic.

- A two-shaded pie chart titled "How was the factor discovered?": It shows the proportion elicited by the clinician versus spontaneously revealed by the patient. Clinicians see that patients usually volunteer the information only about a quarter of the time, which highlights the importance of proactively probing (Figure 7.2, right side).
- A two-shaded pie chart titled "Percentage of contextual factors addressed in the care plan." Like the "Percentage of red flags probed" pie chart, this one shows cumulative performance.
- A bar graph titled "Domains of context": This one shows how contextual factors sort into the 12 domains of context.[2] Just as it's useful for clinicians to see where to look for clues their patients are struggling (contextual red flags), it's useful for them to see where their patients are, in fact, facing challenges that complicate their care. The distribution of contextual factors across the domains of context often seems to reflect sociodemographic

characteristics of the clinic population. For instance, in a low-income population, a high proportion of contextual factors are in the domains of Financial Situation; Access to Care; and Skills, Abilities, and Knowledge. In populations with higher income and educational attainment, contextual factors in the domains of Emotional State, Attitude toward Health Care Provider and System, and Health Behavior may be more predominant (Figure 7.4).

Although these charts and graphs can be compelling, abstractions like "probe rate" and "contextualized POC rate" may not feel meaningful to some clinicians. They need something relatable and concrete. In accordance with the third principle of the QI program—that the value of the project should be evident, as mentioned above—is the 4C format for summarizing examples from recent recorded visits. For instance, a 4C-coded visit is summarized as follows:

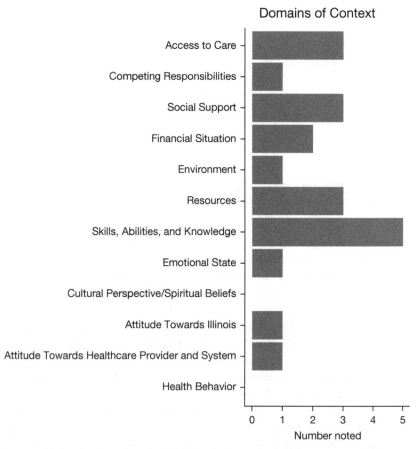

Figure 7.4 Example of 4C data sharing with clinicians about the types and relative frequencies of contextual factors among patients seen at their clinic.

Red flag: The patient missed two appointments that they had scheduled in the past 4 months.

No probe: (The physician never asked why.)

Contextual factor revealed by patient: The patient mentioned having difficulty affording transportation to the VA for appointments.

No contextual POC made: The physician did not acknowledge the patient's comment or suggest potentially helpful VA services, including travel vouchers available through social services.

Examples showing good attention to context included this one:

Red flag: Patient mentions they are not using the CPAP machine to protect their heart and lungs from the effects of sleep apnea.

Probe: The physician asks, "Have you tried it?"

Contextual factor: The patient admits that they have not even opened the package because they heard from a relative that wearing the machine "feels like drowning."

Contextual POC: The physician explains that although some people feel discomfort with the machine, others feel that it really improves their sleep and how they feel the next day. After some discussion, the patient agrees to try the CPAP machine.

Early on, we discovered that examples organized using this format resonate with primary care physicians when shared at their standing clinic meetings because their import is easy to grasp and because the presentation of the information is lean. Key elements are extracted from the noise of the visit, revealing a thread of logic or illogic to those providing the care. The presentations occurred at meetings at which more traditional quality measures are discussed, so they did not seem out of place.

Over time we began to experiment with various ways to provide feedback that were more interactive. For instance, we handed out case examples at standing meetings constructed from recent 4C-coded encounters. Each case contained either a failure to probe a contextual red flag or a failure to incorporate a contextual factor into a care plan. Groups of physicians were given a few minutes to discuss a case, and then we went around asking each to explain why they thought the clinician had overlooked patient context and what they thought could be done differently. Physicians received continuing medical education (CME) credit for participation in these exercises.

After a few such meetings, spaced a month or more apart, we realized that we needed to up the "dose" of feedback and provide more opportunities for physicians to reflect on what they could do differently to improve contextualization of care. Between meetings we started to send out brief e-mail assignments to physicians, which were designed as reflective exercises based on cases from the prior month. Physicians were reminded that completing these exercises would get them CME credit and then, once we got approval, MOC credit from the American Board of

Internal Medicine. About a third completed all or most of the assignments the first year.

A small number of physicians asked us if we could provide them with individualized feedback based on audio recordings of their encounters only. We always agreed to but with the caveat that often we had only a small number of audio recordings for any given physician. It was gratifying, however, to see this level of interest. A couple of physicians explained their interest, saying, "I cringe when I see the aggregate data you provide and I'm wondering if I am part of the problem."

During the first 12 months of the project, 2,583 patients across the Jesse Brown and Hines clinics were approached and invited to participate. Approximately 42% opted in, and, of these, 5% were called in to see their doctor before our project staff had finished introducing them to the project and handing them the audio recorder. So, the overall participation rate was 37%. Consequently, we came away with just under 1,000 audio recordings that first year, involving about 50 physicians. We noticed signs of a dose–response relationship, which refers, in this case, to the change in performance of clinicians in response to differing levels of exposure to the educational interventions. For instance, during the first half-year at Jesse Brown, we invested a lot of time and effort presenting the data at meetings and engaging providers in various reflective exercises both in face-to-face sessions and online. We saw a gratifying improvement in the rate of contextualized care planning from 45% to nearly 70%. That meant that a quarter of the patients whose care depended on addressing factors in their life situation were getting those issues addressed. We started to lose those gains, however, as we diverted our efforts to work on getting the program up and running at Hines Hospital and expanded it to include non-physician providers, as described below. During the final 4 months of the first year of the project at Jesse Brown, we provided no feedback and lost much of our ground; contextualization of care rates fell to 54% by March of 2014.

We observed a similar dose–response relationship at Hines, although the effect was more muted. This may have been, in part, because, for whatever reason, the physicians at Hines started off at a higher baseline level of performance. Interestingly, while we saw improvement in contextualization of care rates at both Jesse Brown and Hines, we had not yet made much of a dent in the lower of the two lines on our graphs—the probing rate. At both sites it sat between 40% and 45% without budging. What does this mean, particularly when overall contextualization of care rates rise? It signifies that physicians are doing a better job at attending to contextual factors that have already been revealed but that they are not improving at noticing and asking about (i.e., probing) contextual red flags. In other words, all the feedback and reflection seemed to heighten their responsiveness to the life challenges they already knew about but did not prompt them to investigate for challenges not yet revealed but for which there were clear hints (i.e., contextual red flags). It is possible that a more intensive program of feedback and reflection would have an effect.

Audit and Feedback as a Physician Nudge

Physicians tell us that the program is a periodic and ongoing reminder of the importance of trying to figure out why a patient seems to struggle with managing their care, nudging them out of making old assumptions. Although we can't know what goes on in the mind of any individual physician as a result of participation, here's an example of what we observe: Dr. Harper is seeing Mr. Anderson for a follow-up exam. Dr. Harper runs down the list of medications that Mr. Anderson is on. Mr. Anderson reports that he is taking his blood pressure medication and a medication for his prostate daily as prescribed. Dr. Harper sees that Mr. Anderson is also supposed to be taking a new cholesterol medication, added at the last visit. He asks, "Are you taking the cholesterol medication?" Mr. Anderson replies that he has never taken it.

In the past, Dr. Harper might have written another prescription for the medication and emphasized the importance of "taking your medicines." He might have written in the notes "non-compliant." But this time, he pauses. Perhaps it was because he had recently been in a discussion with other providers about patient context; perhaps it was because he had discovered from a feedback session that another patient was not taking their medications because they were being stolen from his mailbox. As a result, Dr. Harper stops and asks, "Why aren't you taking it?"

Mr. Anderson explains that he had been instructed to cut the pills in half but that he never received a pill cutter. He went on to say that because he could not cut the pills in half, he did not want to take them incorrectly and so did not take them at all. Dr. Harper was glad he'd asked; this was an easy fix. "If I was able to get you a pill cutter, would you take the medication?" "Sure!"

Mr. Anderson received the right treatment at the right time because his physician thought to elicit and address the underlying context.

Nudging Other Clinicians and Staff

During the early months of the program we only coded data from attending physician–patient encounters. A relatively easy next step was to include residents. The residents who have primary care clinics at Jesse Brown are based in the internal medicine residency program at the University of Illinois at Chicago (UIC) College of Medicine, and those at Hines are from Stritch School of Medicine at Loyola University. In contrast to the attendings, whom we had to court, the residency programs were at once receptive because, fortuitously, we offered a solution to a challenge they faced. The national accreditation organization for internal medicine programs had recently phased in a requirement that all programs incorporate QI activities into their training. Participating in our initiative addressed that requirement.

We began by presenting the program to residents following the approval of their program directors. As a next step, we met with the chief residents. The day-to-day educational activities of large residency programs such as these are managed by chiefs who are just 1 year ahead of the residents in their final year of training. Hence, by engaging and training the chief residents to review and lead feedback exercises on reports, we would no longer need to attend their meetings. We would simply collect and code the data and e-mail them slide decks.

At Jesse Brown, where we trained the chiefs and attended and observed several of their sessions, contextualized care planning rates by residents increased from 50% to 65% over a roughly 9-month period. Our results at Hines lagged compared with Jesse Brown. Hines is 10 miles west in a suburb of Chicago, so we spent much less time there. At Hines, where we trained the chiefs at one session but never directly observed them or had them observe us give feedback, performance actually dropped from 61% to 52%. Because there are so many residents and we had so few coders, the sample sizes behind these numbers were too small to approach statistical significance. But the finding raised the concern that inadequate training of peer facilitators may be counterproductive.

As a next step we expanded the project to include non-physician providers, introducing new challenges. There were several reasons why we had held off on adding nurses, pharmacists, and clerical staff. The first was that we did not want to push the envelope. We thought we would see how things went with just physician participation. Second, we wanted to build trust before expanding to non-physician providers. In particular, we were concerned about how their union stewards would react. We thought that if we could tell them that physicians were already participating and that the staff they represented were already familiar and comfortable with the project (having observed the program as delivered to physicians), there would be less chance of pushback. Finally, the 4C coding system had been developed exclusively from analysis of physician–patient encounters, so we would need to figure out how to adapt it to other types of interactions. What, for instance, constitutes a contextual red flag during an encounter between a veteran and a nurse taking vitals, or a veteran and a clerk, prior to a visit?

Remarkably, the opportunity to expand the program came to us: After one of our presentations at an all-staff team meeting at Jesse Brown, the lead pharmacist asked if we could include clinical pharmacists in the project. Just getting the request was wonderfully encouraging because it provided some affirmation that the project was received, at least by some, in exactly the spirit in which it was intended. If pharmacists wanted to be audio-recorded, it meant that they saw value in the data we provide for their own professional development and felt safe that the information was entirely for their benefit.

It was not difficult to add clinical pharmacists because their role at Jesse Brown is in some respects quite similar to that of primary care physicians. Patients seen in primary care who have complex medication management issues, such as from diabetes or high cholesterol, are often referred to a clinical pharmacist for assistance with medication management. So, when a pharmacist sees a veteran who is struggling to manage their self-care for a chronic condition, our coding team can look for attention to the same contextual issues—red flags and factors—as those that come up during physician visits.

Soon after, we added nurses and clerical staff at Jesse Brown. We started by meeting with their supervisors and then with the union stewards. We did not encounter much resistance. Our timing also was fortunate in that patient-centered care of veterans had become the number one priority for VA leadership nationally. We found that the best way to promote our work was simply to share with people examples of what we were hearing, organized according to the 4C format: contextual red flag, contextual probe, contextual factors, and contextualized care plan.

Once we had support from the unions and managers, we met directly with clerical and nursing staff at their staff meetings. They already knew who we were and what we did. All we had to tell them was that their interactions with patients would similarly be coded and shared for discussion and reflection along with physician encounters. Again, we did not encounter much resistance and even heard rumors of support. The senior nurse manager was particularly enthusiastic.

Including all staff meant that our project team no longer had to restrict participation to veterans in the waiting room who were there to see a physician. If a patient said they were there to see a nurse or a pharmacist, they could now record their visits as well. Adding clerical staff was more of a challenge because it meant intercepting patients as soon as they entered the clinic, before they even got to the front desk, to recruit them and hand them an audio recorder. The licensed practical nurses who completed the initial intake exam, including checking vitals, had always been recorded because every patient passes through a nurse's office or station en route to a doctor visit. So, for that group, it was just a matter of coding rather than ignoring the section of each tape that included this encounter.

Our team began listening to these interactions for the purpose of identifying appropriate contextual red flags and contextual factors. Even when patients check in at the front desk there are opportunities to identify or miss clues that life context is impacting care. For instance, when patients show up 20 minutes or more late for an appointment, they generally are told they will need to wait until after other patients have been seen (and that the provider will have to approve the late visit). But what if the appointment record indicates the patient has been missing or rescheduling appointments repeatedly? Is the clerk asking the patient if there are any particular barriers to getting to their appointments on time? Might it be, for instance, that another time of day would work better, given the veteran's competing responsibilities, such as a work schedule? We soon learned that clerical staff were taught to follow scripts and policies rather than to think contextually, even though there was often a context to the challenges and concerns veterans brought to the front desk. Hence, at subsequent all-staff meetings, we were able to provide feedback with case examples relevant to everyone with whom veterans interact when they come for a visit.

As the project evolved and new ideas came along, we introduced new features to expand the feedback. We added a weekly mass e-mail, for instance, addressed directly from our coders to all providers and staff every Tuesday that, alternatingly, summarizes a recent case example of excellent care and a missed opportunity to address and identify context. The goal is to keep the topic on everyone's minds.

In addition to feedback on contextualization of care, our coders wanted to share with care providers or clerical staff observations that did not fit into the 4C system but seemed too important not to disseminate. In the waiting area, they would hear veterans called for their appointment and then passed over or considered late because they were seated in the wrong location, were hard of hearing, or were too slow to get to the desk before others were called. In the exam room, they would hear frequent disruptions as someone knocked on the door to ask the doctor something or the doctor took a page or answered a phone call in the middle of a discussion with a patient. They noticed that these disruptions sometimes derailed the conversation at a point when the patient was disclosing sensitive information. Some of what they heard was just a startling lack of civility, such as physicians beginning interactions with no greeting or identification. To share these findings, we created an appendix to each report that was printed in blue rather than black font and that gave a variety of examples of things heard on the audio that were critical to patient care but outside of our performance measures. We found these data were often as or more significant in their consequences than the findings in the main report because what our coders heard and shared was so evidently problematic. It was like holding up a mirror and saying, "Have a look. What do you see?" Responsiveness to the "blue" feedback varied. We saw a productive response at an all-staff meeting where participants decided to slide notes under doors rather than knock on them. However, there was no plan to fix the problems identified in the waiting area.

Measuring the Effectiveness of the Audit and Feedback Program

Although we had, up to this point, evidence that contextualization of care is associated with a range of better patient health-care outcomes, we had not yet shown that patient-collected audio with audit and feedback increases rates of contextualization of care among participating providers and, if it does, whether it also improves outcomes. To find that out, we would need research funds to study the program. We had now come full circle: From about 2006 to 2012 we'd conducted basic research, generating the foundational evidence to start the program, which began in 2013. Now, after several years of running the program at two hospital-based clinics, it was time to study its effectiveness.

After several attempts, we were successful at obtaining research funding to study the program. Because research dollars cannot be used to fund QI, we secured a written guarantee from the VISN 12 office that they would cover the QI costs at least until the study was complete. In drafting the proposal, we drew heavily from the young field of implementation science. Implementation science has been described as "the scientific study of methods to promote the systematic uptake of research findings and other evidence-based practices into routine practice, and, hence, to improve the quality and effectiveness of health services and care."[3] Implementation science is characterized by its real-world focus. Just showing that an intervention works is not much use if knowledge is not also acquired about how to integrate it successfully into the health-care environment so that it is effectively implemented.

Combining the study of the effectiveness with the implementation of an intervention is referred to as "hybrid design" in the field of implementation science. We chose a "type 2" design in which equal weight is put on studying effectiveness and implementation. The study involved expanding the audit and feedback QI program to four additional clinics, all within the VA system, located in Milwaukee, Madison, Cleveland, and Los Angeles, in addition to retaining the ones in Chicago and Hines, Illinois. At the new sites, the plan was to begin collecting data at the same time through the introduction of our patient-collected audio recording program but to start providing feedback at different time points at each of the sites, with the rollout randomized by site. This approach to introducing an intervention to clusters of participants at regular intervals is referred to as a "stepped-wedge trial" by implementation scientists. It's similar to a randomized controlled trial in that sites are randomized as to whether they are receiving the intervention versus serving as a control at a point in time. However, it differs in that all sites eventually participate in the intervention.

In addition, we adopted an implementation planning and assessment framework known as RE-AIM, which stands for "reach, effectiveness, adoption, implementation, and maintenance," five components of implementation of a new intervention. As described earlier, we were guided in all our decisions by the three principles of *safety* (i.e., to make providers and patients comfortable with the audio-recording process), *burden* (i.e., to be sure neither feels participating is disruptive to rendering or receiving medical care), and *value* (i.e., to see that they regard participation as worthwhile).

Finally, we designed the study to compare two different levels of intensity of feedback, starting with "standard feedback," which consisted of monthly reports just to primary care providers, and a case-of-the-week e-mailed to all clinical staff. The monthly reports included anonymized case examples that we discussed at standing meetings led by peer clinical champions, nearly all of whom were primary care physicians. Each was trained by our team and supported by a site coinvestigator and a paid research assistant. Clinical champions were respected peers of the participating clinicians at each site. They played a key role at the start of the study, socializing the program to their colleagues and addressing any fears and concerns about the audio recordings and how they would be used. We provided training at a retreat in Chicago for a couple of days before they started.

Standard feedback was followed by "enhanced feedback," in which we expanded the program to include nurses and clinical pharmacists in the same practice groups, residents when present, online reflective exercises for CME and board recertification credit based on the recorded cases, optional individualized reports, and inclusion of data on the outcomes of contextual red flags. When we started the study, Jesse Brown was already providing enhanced feedback, and Hines was providing standard feedback. The other four sites began with baseline data collection without feedback, followed by standard feedback and then enhanced feedback. Figure 7.5 illustrates the stepped-wedge design we employed.

As we launched the study, we realized that we needed a short and pithy name for the program. Over the years we described it variously as "patient-collected audio for audit and feedback to improve contextualization of care" (too long) and the "audit and feedback for contextualizing care intervention package" (suitable only for grant proposals). We decided to call it the Preventing Contextual Errors (PCE) program.

Data collection ran from May of 2017 to May of 2019. Patients were recruited in the waiting rooms, typically by project assistants sitting at a small portable table handing out flyers and putting up posters. Participants were handed small audio recorders. At one site the leadership, under union pressure, mandated that the patients carry the audio recorders out in the open. At the other five sites they would conceal them, although we told patients that if they changed their mind at any point, they could take it out of their pocket or bag or wherever they were hiding it. They could also turn it off if they felt uncomfortable with something being recorded. The latter almost never occurred. When they returned the devices on their way out, we gave them a sticker that said "I helped improve Veterans' care!"

Over 2 years, patients provided us with 4,496 recordings with 666 clinicians. Audio recordings were uploaded to a central server where our 4C team coded them, functioning like a small production line: One member would access the patients' medical records and extract the chart-based red flags, such as missed

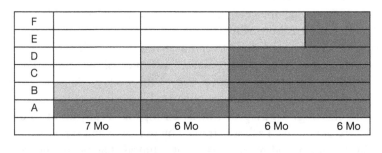

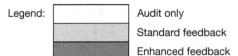

Figure 7.5 Stepped wedge design. The term "audit" refers to the period during which baseline data was collected on contextualization of care rates (at sites C–F) with no feedback to clinicians.
Reprinted from Weiner S, Schwartz A, Altman L, et al. Evaluation of a patient-collected audio audit and feedback quality improvement program on clinician attention to patient life context and health care costs in the Veterans Affairs health care system. JAMA Netw Open. 2020;3(7):e209644.

appointments, low medication refill rates, or frequent emergency department visits. Other members of the team would listen to the audios and extract audio red flags, contextual factors, and contextualized care plans where present. Finally, outcomes were extracted from the medical records several months after the encounter.

This data was then used to produce slide decks for each of the six participating sites, which were e-mailed to the site's clinical champion about every couple of months. Slides were always organized in the same way, beginning with a brief overview of terms and concepts including contextual red flag, contextual probe, contextual factor, and a contextualized care plan. Then we showed them recent examples from their clinic in the following sequence: a missed opportunity to probe a red flag; a missed opportunity to probe a red flag or incorporate a spontaneously revealed contextual factor into a care plan; a red flag probed, eliciting a contextual factor, but with no contextualized POC; a red flag probed but no contextual factor identified (to acknowledge that not all clinical encounters are contextually complex); and, finally, a red flag probed, eliciting a contextual factor that is, in turn, addressed in the POC. Then the slide deck concluded with a run chart, like the one in Figure 7.1. Over time we added more graphics, as described above (Figures 7.2–7.4). These slides were presented at standing meetings.

In the final analysis at the end of the study, we found that 67% of recorded visits contained at least one contextual red flag, of which 55% were probed; 57% of the probes uncovered a contextual factor; and 67% of these contextual factors were addressed in care plans prior to feedback and 72% following feedback, a significant improvement. When we compared standard to enhanced feedback, we didn't see a difference in probing rates; but clinicians were more likely to address contextual factors in their care plans once they were receiving enhanced feedback.

Importantly, we also saw a large and significant effect of contextualization of care on health-care outcomes. Whereas only 46% of non-contextualized care plans had good outcomes (defined as partial or complete resolution of the contextual red flag 4–6 months following the recorded visit), 73% of contextualized care plans had good outcomes. For every six contextual factors identified, a contextualized care plan led to one more improved outcome than expected, a "number needed to treat" of six. If "contextualization of care" were a drug, it would be a blockbuster.

In addition to our analysis of the outcomes of patients who recorded their visits, we looked at how the intervention impacted all of the patients seen by participating clinicians, whether or not they had recorded their visits. After all, if physicians become better at contextualizing care, we should see better outcomes across all their patients. We compared the emergency department visit rates and hospitalization rates of all patients seen by the 666 participating clinicians before and after they received feedback. Once physicians were receiving enhanced feedback, we saw a small but significant decrease in the hospitalization rates of their patients from 19% to 16.5%. This translated to an estimated 987 hospitalizations avoided across the six sites at a cost savings of approximately $25.2 million, based on the cost of an average admission at each site in 2018. The total cost of the intervention, taking into account the personnel time of project assistants and audio coders, was only $337,242, so saving $25.2 million was a return on investment for the intervention of about 75 to 1.

After publishing the findings of the effectiveness of the intervention,[4] we also published a separate report on the implementation process, based on surveys of clinicians and 12 clinician focus groups, surveys of 800 patients, and interviews with 30 facility leaders (five at each site) conducted throughout the study.[5] These sources of data were critical given the novelty, and what some might call intrusiveness, of the intervention. Across all three groups of stakeholders we assessed perceptions of the three design principles of the intervention: Does it feel safe? Is it disruptive or a burden? And do they see value in the program?

Ninety-one percent of patients agreed or strongly agreed with the statement "I feel comfortable recording my visit with my doctor," although some expressed concern that they could be perceived as "spying" on their doctors. Among clinicians, the proportion comfortable with the PCE program was a lower, but still sizeable, majority: 62% strongly agreed or agreed that they felt comfortable with being recorded. In focus groups clinicians often commented that their comfort level with the program grew over time. Fortunately, few patients or clinicians experienced the program as disruptive or burdensome.

Both groups saw the value of the program, with 91% of patients and 75% of clinicians agreeing that the "benefits of the program are clear." Over half of clinicians reported that they found the feedback valuable and that it had changed how they practice. Medical center and clinic leaders expressed especially high levels of enthusiasm in their interviews, with comments such as "I think it's probably long overdue. It's the next generation [of QI]." Some saw the program as a morale booster for clinicians: "It helps them stay excited and engaged about the day-to-day work life" and "I think what's nice about the project is that you really leave it up to the providers to decide how they want to implement it," referring to our philosophy of leaving it to the clinicians to decide how to interpret and use the information. Despite their enthusiasm, however, leaders were noncommittal when asked whether they would fund it with facility resources once the financial support ended.

In sum, we learned that patient-collected audio with audit and feedback can improve contextualization of care, with beneficial downstream effects in terms of both patient-specific outcomes and health-care costs—and that it is well received once participants get used to it.

Despite the effectiveness and appreciation for the program, getting facilities to pay for it proved challenging—and short-lived. Before we had much time to lobby for long-term facility support, the COVID-19 pandemic hit. We were, however, successful in applying for additional research funds to study best approaches to enhancing adoption. Our thought was that if we could bring down the personnel requirements and simplify the protocol, facility leaders might be more inclined to initiate or continue a PCE program. For our program adoption study, we had recruited two new sites—one a large VA medical center ambulatory medicine clinic in Ann Arbor, Michigan, that had not previously participated and the other a large community-based satellite clinic of the Jesse Brown VA Medical Center, where we are based. Jesse Brown had agreed to pay for the QI component of the project. The plan was to test a protocol in which front desk staff would hand out and collect the audio recorders, essentially embedding the program into existing business practices. The goal was to find a way to eliminate the need for designated staff time to recruit patients in the waiting areas.

Even before the pandemic started, however, the prospect that clerical staff would have the time and inclination to add the program to their existing duties may not have been great. It wasn't out of the question, however. In fact, the suggestion came from the director at the community-based satellite clinic, who thought it was feasible. Regardless, everything changed in March of 2020. For several months we suspended all program activity. Then, as we slowly resumed, we had to modify the recruitment protocol to maintain social distancing. Things got a bit easier once vaccination was available, but there was something else we noticed: Patients had lost a lot of their prior sociability. When they came for an appointment, many didn't want to interact with anyone unless doing so was essential to the visit. It became nearly impossible to recruit patients to participate.

At that point we decided to try a different approach. The suggestion came from the director of the community-based clinic we'd added—the same individual who'd suggested before the pandemic that we enlist the assistance of front desk clerks. She suggested we call patients in advance of their appointment to elicit their interest while they were still at home. We sought and obtained approval from the QI committee that had oversight of our program. We also received approval to provide a small incentive in the form of a $10 or $20 gift card, and the Jesse Brown affiliate non-profit foundation agreed to cover the cost.

The impact of these changes was heartening. Many patients responded favorably when contacted in advance of their appointment. Upon reaching patients, it's important to convey that their provider supports the program, that it's fine to say "no thanks" if they are not interested, and that they'll receive a small gift card if they participate (if applicable).

At the time of this writing, 20%–60% of patients reached at home volunteer to record their visit, depending on the clinic and the incentive. Calling patients in advance also substantially reduces the cost of the program because it greatly reduces staff time. It's no longer necessary to have a project assistant hanging out in the waiting room for hours each week. They just show up to meet patients who have already agreed to participate, to equip them with a recorder and collect it when they leave.

The VA maintains a website about the program, designed for those who are interested in adopting it at their clinic.[6] It makes the website accessible to the general public so that it serves as a resource beyond its internal constituencies. Despite the support for the program by senior leadership and its effectiveness, however, the program has a way to go before there is widespread adoption. With the exception of our facility, Jesse Brown VA Medical Center, no site is currently self-financing the program. The reason is quite straightforward, from what we can tell: They don't have to. VA medical centers (and this is equally true of non-VA health systems and practices) already have so many mandates they struggle to follow and fund. Why pay for anything they don't have to?

A rational argument (other than that it improves quality of care and health outcomes) is that it may save money, as we've seen. But for whom? Health systems and hospitals still make money when patients are admitted, so a reduction in admissions may not be financially beneficial. In fact, it could reduce revenue.

Another disincentive is the general discomfort with an audio-recording program despite evidence that it can be accepted and even embraced. Although we've successfully introduced the PCE program to many physicians, clinic directors, and even union stewards, it takes knowledge and experience to do so, which we've acquired over the years. We've found that when enthusiastic colleagues have attempted to start the program at their facility without our close involvement at every step, it stalls, even when the funds are available. And the number of facilities where we have colleagues who are motivated to introduce the program is small. The diffusion of innovation is often a slow and arduous process regardless of the evidence in favor of adoption, particularly when the innovation may seem threatening to some stakeholders.

Legal and Ethical Implications of the PCE Program

When we talk about the PCE program at conferences or other professional meetings, we are sometimes asked about the ethics of covertly recording in the health-care setting or if it is even legal. As described above, legal counsel determined that what we're doing is lawful because clinicians had been informed that they could be recorded. Periodic audio recording as a condition of employment is routine in some other industries. For instance, when callers reach customer service or tech support at many consumer service companies, they hear a recording saying, "This call may be recorded for quality assurance." Employees, in turn, are told something like, "When you work here you will occasionally be recorded while assisting our customers."

So, too, the PCE program. Employees are informed. One difference, however, is that if the recording is started in the waiting room, it might pick up ambient conversations both among staff and between patients or with their families—without their knowledge. In 39 states and on federal property—which includes all VA facilities—it is legal to record conversations if just one party is aware. Any patient at a VA clinic, or any person, for that matter, at health-care facilities in most states, can lawfully turn on the recorder app on their iPhone or other device at any point during their visit without telling anyone.[7] Notably, however, Illinois is one of 11 states that currently require two-party notification. What this means is that we must take precautions to avoid recording parties that have not been notified when employing the same audio-recording methods at UIC just across the street from our VA facility. At UIC, we instruct patients not to turn on their recorders until they are in the exam room with their provider.

A thorny ethical issue is what to do when we hear seriously objectionable behavior by a staff member on an audio recording. On the one hand, we've assured staff that they are safe from any punitive action; on the other, there are some lines they might cross that would obligate us to notify their supervisor. In over a decade of audio recording, this issue has arisen only once. It came up early on when we were first including nurses in the program. Reviewing a recording, our coders heard an intake nurse, whom we'll call "Nurse Draper," ask a veteran if he was participating in the project. Nurse Draper commented that he did not think government should be spying on people. After this occurred, one of us spoke privately with Nurse Draper to share with him what we had heard and tell him that we would welcome discussing with him any concerns that he had. Initially, he asked, "Do I have to participate in this?" and we told him, "Yes," explaining the rationale. We also reiterated how the data is used and not used, particularly stressing that the PCE program has nothing to do with government oversight. We emphasized that if he had any concerns, he should not hesitate to talk with us but never to a patient. At the end of our meeting, he said that he was fine with the project and had no concerns. We thought that would be the end of the matter.

Several weeks later, another veteran, who was accompanied by his wife and had agreed to carry an audio recorder, complained to one of our project staff, Brendan Kelly, that Nurse Draper denied him access to his doctor's appointment because of his participation in our project. The veteran, whom we will call "Roger Meryl," said that after sitting in the waiting area for quite a long time with his hidden audio recorder running, he went up to the front desk to ask about the delay. He was told to talk with Nurse Draper. He went over to Nurse Draper, who said, "I saw you over there talking with that guy with the recorders," pointing to Brendan who had been handing out audio recorders that day. "I called you, but you didn't respond. That was almost an hour ago." Mr. Meryl's wife, standing next to her husband, asked, "So then why didn't you come over and just get us?" Nurse Draper did not reply.

Mr. Meryl came back to his seat and complained to Brendan, who tried to get the veteran in to see his doctor. The physician was available, but Mr. Meryl was already running late for a back-to-back appointment with another provider, so he had to leave without being seen. Our team followed up with him and his wife over the next several days with several phone calls to get his appointment rescheduled.

When our project group met to discuss what to do, we found ourselves in a quandary. On the one hand, we had emphasized the safety aspect of this project, including that we did not report data to supervisors. On the other hand, this was a serious incident resulting in a veteran not getting care at a scheduled appointment and complaining about it. On top of that, there was a political dimension with ramifications potentially at the highest level. Just several weeks earlier a news story had broken nationally that VA medical centers were not truthfully reporting access problems in their clinics. In the worst example, a clinic in Phoenix had a shadow list of veterans who needed appointments but were kept off the official appointment scheduling system so that it appeared that everybody was seen within a month, while, in fact, many waited much longer. The Phoenix incident, and related fallout, led to the resignation of the US secretary of Veterans Affairs. This was not the time to risk a news story that a patient had complained about being barred from access and that we had evidence on tape but took no concrete action.

We started by contacting a trusted senior administrator above the level of Nurse Draper's supervisor. We agreed that one of us would attempt one more time to have an informal conversation with the nurse before making an official complaint. Much to our chagrin, however, whereas Nurse Draper had seemed friendly and open to cooperation after the first meeting, this time he had no apologies and showed no interest in engaging. He said the problem was that our project team in the waiting area was distracting veterans so that they did not know when they were being called. We pointed out to him that during over 1,000 audio-recorded visits a veteran had never missed a visit because of the QI project, but he was not receptive. We told him that if he could not agree to cease interfering with access, we would have to report the situation to his supervisor. He told us we should do whatever we wanted. Having concluded that we had exhausted other options, we notified the nurse manager. She asked for the audio-recorded evidence, so we shared with her the section of the transcript that contained the exchange between the veteran, his wife, and the nurse.

The manager met with Nurse Draper, and because the meeting had potential disciplinary implications, he was invited to include his union representative. We never heard a complaint from the union, but, nevertheless, a rumor spread that we were using the audio recordings to get people in trouble. The first e-mail came from a physician administrator who had supported the project. Her tone was not happy. She seemed concerned that we had done a bait and switch. She is level-headed and pragmatic by temperament; all she needed was the facts. When we explained what occurred, she was reassured and responded that we had done the right thing.

At the next all-staff meeting, after we had finished presenting the latest round of data as feedback, a physician who rarely spoke up at meetings did so. In an angry tone, he said that we were using the project to report staff to their supervisors and that this was not what he and others had been told would occur. Several other staff chimed in, adding their concern. We explained that the circumstances that led to our report to a supervisor were such that we felt we had no choice and had exhausted other options. In responding, we were cautious about sharing details, given that this was a personnel matter and should not be traceable to a particular individual. Nurse Draper was sitting at a table near the front, the first time we had seen him at a meeting.

We stressed several points, first, that the incident began with a veteran complaining about how he had been treated, not with our responding to something we heard on audiotape. In other words, the audio was used only to corroborate a veteran's complaint. Second, we pointed out that our original promise not to disclose performance data for any participant with their supervisor still held. The information that we disclosed was not performance data. It had nothing to do with contextual red flags or contextual factors. It was evidence of an employee undermining a patient's access to care. Third, we noted that the subject matter of the particular complaint—access to care—was one that the VA could not afford to disregard. Finally, we added that, prior to reporting the nurse to a supervisor, we had made several attempts to speak with him directly.

Nurse Draper raised his hand and asked who had the transcripts. His voice was calm and matter-of-fact; there was no indication that he was the staff member we were all talking about. Playing along, we replied that the transcripts were in the hands of the supervisor of the individual in question. At that point, the physician who so vociferously opposed the project spoke up saying that he did not think we should have shared the audio transcripts. He said we should have just forwarded the complaint but without disclosing what was on the audio. At that point Nurse Draper's supervisor, who was also in the room, spoke up to defend the project and our reporting of the incident. She said she had the transcripts, that the nurse had not behaved appropriately, and that she discussed it with that person.

We closed by saying we would take the concerns raised to the quality committee overseeing the project. The physician who initiated the discussion asked skeptically who was on the committee. We mentioned that the committee had representation from each of the stakeholder groups. After the meeting, an influential primary care physician who is respected for being evenhanded, helpful, and knowledgeable about how things work in the VA system came over to indicate that he had "no problem" with the project. An advanced practice nurse e-mailed one of us later that morning to say she was concerned, but when we followed up with a phone call and shared the particulars of why we reported the incident, she, too, was supportive. She made the helpful analogy that using audio to corroborate an allegation seems comparable to a surveillance camera corroborating an allegation. Surveillance cameras are not there to spy on employees. They are there for security purposes. But were a veteran to complain that an employee had attacked them in the presence of a camera, there is no reason to think administrators would not or should not look at what was captured on video.

We contacted the director of QI, who also sits on the quality committee. She referred the case to the hospital ethics committee. The director of the ethics committee at the time was a psychiatrist who routinely provides consultation on the care and management of hospitalized patients. Ethicists are often called when a care team, the patient, and/or their family cannot agree on a care plan. They are accustomed to tense, difficult situations. Our case was distinctly unusual, however, given that it did not involve a particular patient's care. The ethics committee had not been aware of our project and said they knew little about the ramifications of audio-recording staff. They said they would review the case but also wanted a consultation from legal counsel about the incident.

Because the lawyer who had originally approved the project had left, we spoke with another attorney assigned to the VA facility. Legal counsel arrived at essentially the same conclusion as the nurse who compared audio to a surveillance camera. The attorney said that we are obligated to report evidence that an employee is "harming" a veteran regardless of whether we see it directly with our eyes or come upon it through the medium of technology. She also pointed out that the use of the transcripts to corroborate the allegations of the veteran was protective of the employee as well as the veteran. We could have just as easily found, from listening to the audio, that the patient's allegations were not substantiated by the audio.

The ethics committee endorsed the opinion of legal counsel. The incident, while unfortunate, brought to the fore the question of when to disclose identifiable data from audio to employees' supervisors. The conclusion of the legal and ethics oversight bodies was that the same standard should apply whether observing misconduct seen in real time or captured inadvertently through technology. And while we'd used the recording to substantiate a complaint first made by a veteran, we'd be obligated to report an incidentally observed case of misconduct, even in the absence of a complaint. The message to those wary of being audio-recorded is that the expectations for good behavior are no different from those in all encounters with patients.

USPS FOR AUDIT AND FEEDBACK

While analysis of real patient encounters is likely to remain at the center of performance assessment of attention to patient life context in care planning, USPs can play a distinct niche role. As illustrated in research described in Chapter 2, USPs can be scripted to assess a wide range of performance characteristics, enabling targeted feedback. If, for instance, you are concerned that a group of physicians are not addressing poor patient medication adherence, you can train USPs to present with adherence barriers, collect data on clinician performance when seeing just a few of these (fake) patients, and then share the findings with them. The intervention can be structured as a plan–do–study–act cycle.

Of course, setting up USP visits is complicated and incurs costs. They are paid employees, or subcontractors, of the QI team and require training. Setting up the subterfuge so that they appear authentic to providers is an elaborate process. One also must address various concerns that physicians, practice administrators, and others may raise. For instance, some object to USPs on the grounds that they displace the care of real patients by taking their appointment slots. However, in truth, the effect is miniscule. For instance, Hines VA Medical Center has about 800,000 outpatient visits per year, and we scheduled about 130 USP visits over 2 years, displacing 0.008% of appointments.

Although we began our research on contextualization of care by utilizing USPs to collect data on clinician performance, employing them as a strategy to *improve* performance came late in our work. An opportunity arose outside the VA through our company, the Institute for Practice & Provider Performance Improvement, or I3PI. We first got the idea for I3PI during our first USP study when several clinic directors asked us if we could share our data so that they could see which of their physicians were excelling and which were doing poorly. Of course, we said "no" as that would have violated the terms of the informed consent process. As a result of these requests, however, we realized that we did in fact have a service of value.

These clinic directors knew that a lot happens in the exam room when the door is closed that distinguishes clinicians who are doing a great job from those who just look like they are from their notes. The problem they recognized is a gap in how quality is measured. Clinician performance is currently assessed based on what's in the medical record and from patients' reported experiences on surveys. What's missing is a window into what actually occurs during the medical encounter. The exam room is a black box. We started I3PI to help practices look into that black box and improve the value of the care their physicians were providing.

From the beginning, we found it slow-going. It's one thing for practice managers to ask for data informally from a project their practice isn't paying for and another to spend money for a service that could reveal problems they weren't mandated to address. And at the start, we didn't have evidence that sharing data collected from USP visits could change practice and whether such changes would save enough money to justify the costs of a USP program.

I3PI partnered with the American College of Physicians and approached the Robert Wood Johnson Foundation (RWJF) for funding to gather that evidence. First, we needed to identify a health systems partner that would work with us. We eventually partnered with Horizon Blue Cross Blue Shield of New Jersey. The RWJF provided the funds to cover the costs of our and our staff's time and the training and deployment of actors recruited primarily from standardized patient programs and theater communities in the New Jersey area. Based on Horizon's QI priorities at the time, we developed four USP case scripts designed to assess behaviors of physicians in primary care practices seeing patients with diabetes, opioid requests for chronic back pain, evidence of depression, tobacco use, and indications for cancer screening. When designing the checklists for each case we focused on clinically significant performance characteristics that can only be assessed through direct observation. For instance, it requires direct observation to distinguish between a physician who just says to a patient who smokes "you really should quit" and one who also assesses their readiness to quit and discusses cessation medications and effective strategies. Both might document that they "counseled patient on smoking cessation," but only the latter has employed an approach that has been demonstrated to be more effective.

The scope of the RWJF study was broader than testing whether USPs can improve contextualization of care. We wanted to see if USPs could improve overall quality, including reducing overuse and misuse of medical services. Included in the scripts we wrote were contextual red flags and contextual factors. For instance, in one case a young woman had developed erratic diabetes control (a contextual red flag) since starting a relationship with a young man. The contextual factor was that she'd been uncomfortable telling him about her medical condition. In another, poor diabetes control (red flag) followed loss of coverage for the long-acting insulin the patient was taking (contextual factor). In a third, a patient declined cervical cancer screening (red flag) because she thought this kind of cancer couldn't be prevented (contextual factor). And in a fourth, a patient declined colon cancer screening (red flag) also because they didn't think it worth going through the procedure (contextual factor).

An advantage of USPs for assessing contextualization of care is that you already know what the contextual red flags and factors are. You just need to make checklists of what would count as contextualized care for each script to score clinician performance. We intentionally set the bar quite low to give credit for any observable effort by a clinician to attend to patient context. For instance, any conversation with the young woman about her social anxieties about her diabetes diagnosis counted, or a referral to a psychologist with patient consent.

Twenty-two practices across New Jersey agreed to participate. Of the 64 providers at these practices, 59 consented to the protocol. We set up the study such that each clinician would receive two USP visits at baseline followed by two USPs after feedback. Following each USP visit, actors completed checklists online and uploaded their audio recordings. Our team validated the checklists based on the audios and completed checklists based on the physicians' notes to determine whether the final plan was contextualized. We e-mailed individual reports to each provider and an aggregate report to each practice summarizing the findings for participating clinicians. Reports benchmarked providers' performance against the average of their peers. After sending the report, one of us would meet (virtually) with the clinicians at a practice to go over the findings and discuss an intervention plan. For instance, a practice might learn that none of them discussed smoking cessation medication options, whereas 25% of their peers did. They might also learn that only three of the five of them (slightly higher than their peers but still not that good) both identified the reasons why this young patient was not taking her diabetes medication (i.e., the contextual factor) and then addressed those reasons in their care plan (i.e., contextualized the care plan). To address the former finding, we'd send them a review article on evidence-based tobacco cessation counseling and management and, to address the latter, a handout on the 12 domains of life context to consider in the setting of medication non-adherence—and ask how they planned to change their approach to managing these clinical situations.

After the feedback sessions, we sent each practice USPs with different clinical presentations but with the same performance assessment characteristics. So, for instance, the practice above would get USPs who smoked and had barriers to taking their medications. We could then assess whether the clinicians were more effective using the same scoring criteria employed in the baseline measures.

The intervention was effective in some areas assessed.[8,9] Significant improvement areas included smoking cessation counseling, managing chronic low back pain without opioids, and depression screening. But we did not see improvements in addressing contextual factors, such as financial barriers, patients' anxieties, and misunderstandings that accounted for low medication adherence or participation in cancer prevention screening.

When comparing the lack of effectiveness of the USPs to the effectiveness of real patient-collected audio at improving contextualization of care, it should be noted that USP feedback was provided only once rather than on an ongoing basis. Furthermore, the real patient intervention focused exclusively on improving contextualization of care, whereas the USP program was broader, potentially diluting the emphasis on addressing patient life context in care planning.

In addition to assessing the impact of feedback on the care of fake patients, we wanted to see whether audit and feedback with USPs changed the way the clinicians cared for their real patients. After all, if our intervention is changing how clinicians practice, we should detect those changes across their entire practice, not just with the fake patients we send them. Because real patient visits were not recorded, we looked at claims data provided by Horizon for all patients seen at the participating practices both before and after we provided feedback to clinicians. We obtained concurrent claims data from a similar group of practices that did not participate in the study for comparison.

Better care is not necessarily cheaper care, at least within the short window of time we were looking at. For instance, improving medication adherence in patients with diabetes by addressing contextual factors should reduce costs as there are likely fewer visits, fewer referrals, and so on. In contrast, improving cancer screening in patients who were previously reluctant to get a colonoscopy or mammogram actually generates more claims for these procedures (even though in the long run it should reduce costs of cancer care).

Overall, per-visit claims went up across the board in both the intervention and control groups, consistent with the rising costs of health care. Adjusting for these external effects, however, changes in claims costs occurred as would be expected with better care. For instance, claims for cancer screening went up more in the intervention than comparison group for real patients during the period after clinicians in the intervention group received USP feedback. They also went up for smoking cessation–related claims. Conversely, they went down for office-based diabetes care.

A limitation of claims data, however, is that we couldn't always determine exactly what kinds of care the patients were receiving, only whether the rates of claims were changing. As a result, in contrast to the real patient study, the USP study did not as affirmatively demonstrate effectiveness. That does not mean that USP audit and feedback is a weaker intervention. The fact that we saw an effect with just one round of feedback suggests that it might even be more potent than audit & feedback with real patients. USPs provide a penetrating assessment because they are customized to target specific quality concerns, also with direct observation. And, although they may seem more costly, that is not definitively the case.

The most striking example is the change in care to the patients with diabetes: The marginal cost of two USP visits to a provider (i.e., not counting the fixed costs of setting up the program) was approximately $700, and 110 of these were scripted to facilitate better diabetes care. That's $77,000, which is not cheap. However, we saw a difference-in-difference claims cost reduction of $54.08 across 58,479 visits by patients with diabetes, a cost reduction of $3.2M. If these cost savings were, in fact, for better care, it would be penny-wise and pound-foolish not to employ USPs widely.

CDS TO FACILITATE CONTEXTUALIZATION OF CARE

A general limitation of audit and feedback, whether from real patient or USP visits, is that it can only affect future care. CDS, in contrast, utilizes technology to guide clinicians in real time during the clinical encounter. CDS draws on patient-specific data in the electronic medical record (e.g., how old a patient is, what medications they are taking, what medical conditions they have) to influence clinician decision-making at the point of care. CDS is commonly utilized to remind clinicians, for instance, when a patient is due for a colonoscopy or mammogram, needs a flu vaccine, or should avoid certain medications because of drug interactions or allergies. Might it also improve contextualization of care?

In 2017 we received funding from the Agency for Healthcare Research and Quality to develop and test some ideas we had for configuring CDS to guide clinicians to contextualize care. The basic design has two elements. First, patients can complete a questionnaire before their visit in the patient portal that explicitly probes for common contextual red flags as well as eliciting less common ones with an open-ended query. Any positive responses prompt follow-up questions to elicit contextual factors across the 12 contextual domains. These will pre-populate the clinician's electronic note at the start of the visit. For instance, the first probe reads "Are you having difficulty taking medications the way you have been told to take them?" If the patient selects "yes," they are given a list of possible reasons (i.e., contextual factors) to choose from. If they select, for instance, "My medication is too expensive" (which is in the contextual domain of "financial situation"), that response will appear in a "contextual care box" in the template at the start of the visit, just like the patient's problem list, medication list, and vital signs.

Second, CDS tools scan the patient's medical record for common contextual red flags, such as missed appointments, not refilling medication, and loss of control of a chronic condition, also to pre-populate the clinician's note. Each red flag has a specific threshold that triggers sending the information into the contextual care box. For instance, if the glycated hemoglobin had increased by more than 1% since the prior measurement, that would trigger notification to the clinician as a statement that "Your patient has a glycated hemoglobin that has risen by >1%." These thresholds were taken directly from our 4C coding manual because we had previously determined that they should prompt a clinician to consider whether their patient is facing some sort of life challenge (contextual factor) that warrants contextual probing.

In addition to pre-populating the clinician's note at the start of the visit with contextual red flags and factors elicited from the patient and culled from the medical record, the CDS tools were designed to suggest some logical next steps. For instance, when a patient has loss of health insurance coverage, a referral to the facility's indigent care office pops up. The clinician can, at that point, accept or ignore the order. If they accept the order, a phrase goes into their note indicating that the patient was referred to the indigent care office. We used these pop-ups sparingly to avoid alert fatigue. Figure 7.6 provides a schematic of the overall

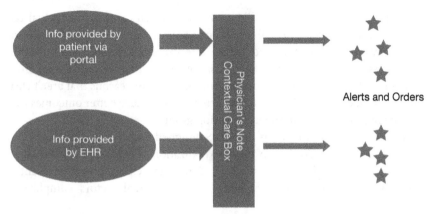

Figure 7.6 Contextual information (factors and red flags) noted by patients or harvested from information in the medical record is aggregated into a "contextual care box" in physician's note and, when warranted, activates alerts and orders. EHR = electronic health record.

design, intended to show how information coming from the patient and information coming from their medical record are routed into the physician's note and, concurrently, utilized to activate various alerts and orders.

We conducted a randomized controlled trial to see whether our "contextualized CDS" as we called it, changed clinician practice (by increasing contextualization of care) and improved patient health-care outcomes. We defined "improved patient health-care outcomes" as we had in our prior studies: as partial or full resolution of the presenting contextual red flag. So, if the glycated hemoglobin had gone up by 2%, as noted at the index visit, we considered any reduction at 4–6 months following the index encounter an improvement.

We designed the CDS to function in both Epic and Cerner, two widely utilized electronic medical records, and recruited patients at sites employing both systems. Four hundred and fifty-two patients consented to carry concealed audio recorders into their visit. Prior to their visits they completed the questionnaire. Patients didn't know whether they were in the control or intervention group. If they were in the control, their questionnaire responses never went into the contextual care box and the CDS never culled data from the electronic health record. As a result, the clinician got no contextual information about the patients from the CDS and no guidance.

Because visits were audio-recorded in both the intervention and control, we were able to code them to see whether clinicians were probing for context at different rates in the two groups. Our 4C coders didn't know at the time of coding whether they were listening to a control or an intervention visit. They also didn't know 4–6 months later when they checked the outcomes of the contextual red flags.

As described in our publication of the study,[10] the intervention significantly increased both contextual probing and contextualization of the care plan. Although contextual red flags were not more likely to resolve in the intervention versus the control arm, they were more likely to resolve when care was contextualized, *regardless of study arm*. These findings may seem counterintuitive. If care was more likely to be contextualized in the intervention arm and contextualized care was associated with better outcomes, how was it that we didn't see a larger number of better outcomes in the intervention arm? For reasons that aren't clear, contextualized care plans in the control arm tended to have better outcomes than contextualized care plans in the intervention group.

Regardless, what we can say is that CDS designed to draw clinicians' attention to patient life context can improve contextualization of care. And contextualization of care, as seen in both prior studies and this one, helps resolve the presenting indicators that patients are struggling with contextual factors complicating their care.

In addition to recruiting real patients to record their visits for the CDS study, we employed USPs to assess the impact of the CDS, in large part because USP scripts could be customized around the CDS features we sought to assess. Thus, we needed only a few USP visits to test the intervention because every visit would activate a number of CDS effects. In addition, with USP visits, we could make apples-to-apples comparisons between intervention and control visits.

For this part of the study, we wrote scripts for four different USPs, designed to test the effectiveness of various features of the contextualized CDS we had designed. For instance, one USP presented as a heavyset woman in her forties with a history of sleep apnea, poorly controlled diabetes and hypertension, and depression, who complains of recent fatigue. She is caring for two young children while also working the night shift at a factory. On a pre-visit questionnaire in the patient portal, she discloses that her CPAP machine is broken, that one of her diabetes medications (dulaglutide) is too expensive, and that she sometimes forgets to take her medication, in part because she feels overwhelmed and sad much of the time. During an intervention visit, these responses appeared in the contextual care box in the note template, so the clinician saw them right away. In addition, the CDS would generate a referral order to the sleep lab. During control visits, of course, none of the information appeared and no actions were automated. The clinician was, as usual, on their own when it came to eliciting relevant patient context and deciding what to do in the control visits.

When we designed this part of the study, we planned to do 80 USP visits. Each of the four scripts would be portrayed at 10 control visits without CDS support and 10 intervention visits with CDS support, divided across the two sites. However, midway through, the COVID-19 pandemic started, so we were forced to stop data collection after just 41 visits. Protecting the safety of our actors and participating clinicians necessitated ending this component of the study.

Despite the small sample size, there were still some significant and interesting findings. Foremost is that intervention encounters were more than twice as likely to have contextualized care plans than control encounters. This reinforces the results with real patients and was not surprising to us given that the CDS was highly active during intervention visits because the scripts were designed to trigger multiple prompts. Unlike the real patient visits, however, probing rates were not higher in intervention USP visits. The improvement in contextualization of care despite low probing rates points to a unique benefit of the CDS design: By eliciting contextual factors as well as red flags and proposing interventions based on those factors, it reduces some of the need to probe. So, for instance, even if a physician neglects to probe the USP's comment that she has been tired more lately, the CDS in the intervention arm makes it easy to do the right thing. First, the physician will learn that their patient has stopped using her CPAP machine because it's broken, even if the physician never asked. And if they ignore that information, they'll see suggested orders to refer the patient to have the equipment repaired that they merely need to sign. Contextualized CDS makes it harder to do the wrong thing—to miss an opportunity to contextualize care.

KEY POINTS

- Improving actual performance in practice at contextualization of care, rather than just skill (i.e., narrowing the "skills-to-performance" gap), can be achieved through both audit and feedback, in which clinicians learn from past experience to improve future practice, and CDS, in which they are nudged to attend to patient context in real time during the medical encounter.
- One effective approach to audit and feedback utilizes patient-collected audio: Patients record their visits, the data is analyzed utilizing 4C, and the results are shared with clinicians. A VA program utilizing patient-collected audio with recurring feedback was associated with significantly increased contextualization of care (against a control), with a greater likelihood of improved outcomes and with estimated cost savings that were vastly in excess of the costs of the intervention.
- Another approach to audit and feedback utilizes USPs (or fake patients) to record visits: In a community-based study of primary care practices, a comparison of the care of USPs before versus after clinician feedback (and adjusted against a control) did not increase contextualization of care. A major difference from the patient-collected audio program, however, is that clinicians received feedback just once. Remarkably, however, it did improve overall quality of care, including smoking cessation counseling and management of lower back pain and depression. Also, there was evidence that the effect carried over to the care of these clinicians' real patients based on an analysis of claims of patients pre- versus post-intervention (also adjusted against a control). It even appeared to improve the contextualization of care of these real patients, with substantial cost savings.
- Contextualized CDS improved both contextual probing and contextualization of care in a randomized controlled trial. However,

while contextualization of care continued to predict improved health-care outcomes (defined as partial or full resolution of the contextual red flag), we were not able to establish that our contextualized CDS independently improves health-care outcomes.

NOTES

1. Binns-Calvey AE, Sharma G, Ashley N, Kelly B, Weaver FM, Weiner SJ. Listening to the patient: a typology of contextual red flags in disease management encounters. J Patient Cent Res Rev. 2020;7(1):39–46.

2. Binns-Calvey AE, Malhiot A, Kostovich CT, et al. Validating domains of patient contextual factors essential to preventing contextual errors: a qualitative study conducted at Chicago area Veterans Health Administration sites. Acad Med. 2017;92(9):1287–1293.

3. Eccles MP, Mittman BS. Welcome to *Implementation Science*. Implement Science. 2006/02/22 2006;1(1):1.

4. Weiner S, Schwartz A, Altman L, et al. Evaluation of a patient-collected audio audit and feedback quality improvement program on clinician attention to patient life context and health care costs in the Veterans Affairs health care system. JAMA Netw Open. 2020;3(7):e209644.

5. Ball SL, Weiner SJ, Schwartz A, et al. Implementation of a patient-collected audio recording audit & feedback quality improvement program to prevent contextual error: stakeholder perspective. BMC Health Serv Res. 2021;21(1):891.

6. Department of Veterans Affairs. Preventing Contextual Errors program. https://marketplace.va.gov/innovations/preventing-contextual-errors-pce-program. Last accessed June 16, 2022.

7. Schwartz A. Toward a patient right to record medical visits. UIC Law Review. 2023;57(1).

8. Schwartz A, Peskin S, Spiro A, Weiner SJ. Impact of unannounced standardized patient audit and feedback on care, documentation, and costs: an experiment and claims analysis. J Gen Intern Med. 2021;36(1):27–34.

9. Schwartz A, Peskin S, Spiro A, Weiner SJ. Direct observation of depression screening: identifying diagnostic error and improving accuracy through unannounced standardized patients. Diagnosis. 2020;7(3):251–256.

10. Weiner SJ, Schwartz A, Weaver F, et al. Effect of electronic health record clinical decision support on contextualization of care: a randomized clinical trial. JAMA Network Open. 2022;5(10):e2238231.

8

What We Can't Measure
That Matters

> "Not everything that can be counted counts, and not everything that counts can be counted."
>
> —WILLIAM BRUCE CAMERON[1]

There is a dimension to contextualizing care that flies under the radar of what we code but is nevertheless foundational to effective care. It has to do with the clinician's capacity to employ themselves as the intervention when the context is something that a patient is thinking or feeling. Recall that six of the 12 domains of patient context (i.e., the ones on the right side of Table 1.1) pertain to drivers of behavior, including a patient's emotional state, their cultural perspective/spiritual beliefs, their attitude toward their illness, and their attitude toward their health-care provider and system. When a patient has missed appointments, has not taken their medication, or exhibits hostile behavior toward their doctor and the context is that they are angry, distrustful, anxious, or feel humiliated, the clinician's response can have a huge impact on subsequent behavior.

We present here an extended case example that illustrates the complexity of employing one's self effectively as the intervention in the care of a patient whose emotional state is complicating their care. The contextual red flag in the case is a patient's dysfunctional behavior at appointments. There are a range of possible approaches to eliciting the underlying context (i.e., contextual probing) and addressing it (i.e., contextualizing care), but 4C isn't designed to discern among them. Nevertheless, how the clinician responds may be extremely important to the patient's care.

CASE EXAMPLE

When the physician opened David Mason's chart in a Veterans Affairs (VA) clinic just before an appointment, a "behavioral warning flag" popped up that read, "Mr. Mason has had multiple incidents of verbal and physical abuse of staff and other patients; he also made a serious threat against staff. Avoid caring for the patient in secluded areas. If Veteran does not respond to de-escalation and verbal redirection by staff, call VA police." Mr. Mason, 56 years old and 6 feet tall, had been coming to the medical center for 20 years, since 1996. He was scheduled with a new physician after a previous doctor refused to care for him any longer. The final straw had been that the patient, angry that his physician would not prescribe narcotics, commented during a visit to the emergency room (ER) requesting hydrocodone that he could kill his doctor for not giving him what he needed. The ER informed the physician of the incident. The physician said he would not see the patient again. Today was the patient's first visit to a new primary care doctor. Several months had passed since Mr. Mason was last prescribed opioids, according to an online state database.

What was most striking about reviewing the 2,724 notes written about Mr. Mason over two decades was how little information was contained within them. Among hundreds of notes by primary care physicians, social workers, psychiatrists, and case managers, there were just a few facts about his life, typically copied and pasted from one record to the next. Mr. Mason was born and raised in Chicago and lived with four sisters and two parents. His dad suffered from depression and alcoholism. A note mentioned that for a part of his childhood he had been sent south of the city to live with a grandmother to keep him out of the reach of gangs. He'd finished the 11th grade; served in the Marines for a year, with no combat exposure; and then left with an honorable discharge after a training accident on an obstacle course resulted in a herniated disc. For about 8 years, he worked in maintenance for the Chicago Housing Authority. His life since had been chaotic, with two failed marriages, domestic abuse, alcoholism, cocaine abuse, two prison terms for burglary, and two suicide attempts with pill overdoses. Many of these life events were documented in real time as they played out during his years coming to VA medical centers. Perusing through thousands of notes, one caught fragments of events as they occurred. His first prison term, for instance, was registered as a 2.5-year gap in the chart. He had not come in for visits, and the first note upon his return simply said he was away in prison.

New hardships hit. He lost all three of his adult children: A 26-year-old daughter had been raped and murdered the prior summer. Before that, a 37-year-old daughter had died of an overdose. A 21-year-old son was shot and killed. The physician noted that Mr. Mason's first opioid prescriptions coincided with these deaths and had increased following the loss of his youngest child.

Three VA police officers were called to stand by as Mr. Mason was led into the exam room. They stood outside with bulletproof vests, noisy walkie-talkies, and pistols as the attending physician and a resident shut the door to the exam room. After introducing himself and the resident, the attending set the stage:

Mr. Mason, I'm sorry to have the police just outside the door but I understand from the chart that you've threatened people and there is a notice saying we must have the police stand by. I also understand that you've been frustrated about other doctors not giving you narcotics for your pain. Can you tell me about the pain you are having?

The opener was direct, the elephant in the room named: that there are police guarding the two physicians and that the patient has had a specific agenda in the past. And then, without pause, the physician followed up with a question that demonstrated he was not skirting the patient's concern. In fact, it was the first thing he wanted to talk about. The doctor demonstrated matter-of-fact directness combined with caring. His body language reinforced both: He positioned himself, seated at eye level, just a couple of feet away from the veteran, with full eye contact, focused and calm.

Mr. Mason ignored the question and launched into a litany of complaints about VA doctors not helping him get the Norco (hydrocodone with acetaminophen) that he needs and saying he wanted it immediately. The attending, who was not surprised by the outburst, responded by putting his cards on the table, replying that he would like to help with any medical issues, including pain, but that there were reasons he would not prescribe a narcotic. First was that the patient had cocaine in several urine drug tests. The doctor explained that cocaine can be laced with synthetic opioids and explained the dangers. To prescribe narcotics to a patient under such circumstances carried additional risk, and he was not willing to take that risk. The doctor was intentional in framing his response in terms of what risk he was willing to take rather than the patient's risk tolerance because he knew that the latter could be turned back on him. He'd had other patients say, essentially, "Well, I'm willing to take the risk." Second, the attending commented that several urine tests did *not* show expected levels of prescribed narcotics, raising the question of whether he'd been giving some of the medicine to other people. While conveying this information, he was aware that he was wielding power over his patient, which he regretted but also felt was necessary.

Mr. Mason shifted from bullying to pleading: "Doc, I know I've made mistakes, but I'm in pain and you've got to help me." "Show me where it's hurting," the physician replied, while coming closer. Mr. Mason pointed to several areas including his back, his hand, and a leg. The physician examined each body part carefully, taking the veteran's hand in his as he looked and gently palpated the areas that he was told hurt. While he examined Mr. Mason, he asked him questions about how long he'd had these pains. Then he asked where he lived, and Mr. Mason said he'd been on the streets. He said he avoided shelters because they were violent and dirty, preferring to sleep outdoors. He talked about some of the places where he felt safe and warm. The physician commented that upon reviewing the medical record he saw that a social worker who has been following Mr. Mason's case had noted that they seemed close to getting him housed through a special program for veterans experiencing homelessness. The doctor asked Mr. Mason, "How optimistic are you that this is all going to work out in the next couple of weeks?" Mr.

Mason replied, "I'm really not convinced." The doctor said, "Let's see if we can reach the social worker," and picked up the phone. There was no answer, so he left a message. He also sent an e-mail while the patient watched.

During the visit, the conversation expanded. Mr. Mason brought up the deaths of his three adult children. He talked about his remorse that he has been such a bad example to his family. He described how his grief at the death of his children was compounded by guilt and said that he was trying to provide good care to his grandchildren, for whom he now had a lot of responsibility. They were scattered about, but he said that he kept a close eye on them and noted that when he had his own place, he would become more involved.

What stood out to the physician during the conversation was the coherence of Mr. Mason's thought processes and use of language. He did not say things that were unnecessary or tangential. His responses to questions were concise. He spoke using sentence structure correctly despite a relatively low level of education. He was open about himself and direct. He seemed highly intelligent. The physician also noted his capacity for self-insight. He thought about bringing up his concerns that Mr. Mason might be medicating himself with opioids to manage his grief but thought that mentioning the word might trigger him to start demanding them again. Instead, he commented that Mr. Mason was coping with a lot of stress and grief and suggested a referral for counseling. Mr. Mason responded that he'd tried that before and that it never did anything for him. He wasn't interested.

As the attending was wrapping up the encounter, Mr. Mason demanded narcotics again. It was as if, seeing the end of the visit approaching, he reacted as though someone had thrown a switch. Calm, thoughtful discussion changed to indignation, agitation, and an assertion that if he could not have narcotics there was no point being there. He said he would have to get himself another doctor. He looked hurt and angry. However, he never seemed threatening. He got up and stormed out. The attending noted, however, a slight reluctance in his gait as he left, suggesting that something about the encounter made him ambivalent about leaving. He made a note to himself to call the patient later to check on him. When the doctor did call, it went to voicemail. He left a message saying he looked forward to seeing him at his next visit.

A few weeks later, Mr. Mason showed up for a scheduled follow-up. This time the doctor called for just a single police officer. He greeted Mr. Mason in the waiting area and ushered him back into the exam room. He noticed an unexpected feeling in himself. Whereas he had some apprehension awaiting the encounter, as soon as he saw Mr. Mason and began to interact with him, it was replaced with a warm anticipation, a sense that this man could engage with him. He felt glad to see him.

The appointment started out with the expected demand for opioid medication. The doctor thought about how this dynamic had affected Mr. Mason's care. Looking at prior notes, it was striking how often these outbursts had crowded out nearly everything else. Mr. Mason had diabetes, for which he took medications, yet no one had checked a glycated hemoglobin in 2 years; he had heart disease, yet no one had checked his lipids. Mr. Mason, through disruptive behavior, sabotaged the physician-patient relationship. Could this be the point? Pushing his doctors away, while counterproductive to his health, could be the functional and self-protective response of a Black man who has experienced racism and judgment from too many providers. Perhaps he'd concluded that the only thing of value he got from these appointments were narcotics, and he only received those through bullying and cajoling.

The doctor decided to pick up where he'd left off at the last visit. He said he remembered the housing issues he'd talked about and wondered how things were going. Mr. Mason replied that he now had an apartment and that it was a big relief. He said it didn't come with much furnishing or bedding, however, and that he was having trouble getting clean and insect-free secondhand items. He discussed the places he had tried, including the Salvation Army and a VA basement warehouse that serves veterans experiencing homelessness. During the conversation, Mr. Mason mentioned that although he was glad to have a place of his own, the grief he felt at the loss of his children and the mistakes he had made went with him everywhere, whether on the streets or in an apartment. The doctor asked about suicide risk. Mr. Mason replied that because he wanted to be there for his grandkids, he did not feel he was at risk of hurting himself. The conversation shifted to his various health issues. The doctor said he was concerned about Mr. Mason's diabetes and heart condition and would like to discuss those and see what he could do.

Just as it seemed the visit was on track, Mr. Mason returned to his cry for narcotics. Again, that switch had flipped. He insisted—his voice rising—that there was no point staying if he could not get Norco and that he needed another doctor. He got up and exited as he had after the first visit. The attending wondered, as he watched Mr. Mason stumble out, whether he might be running away from something he feared. Could he fear the risks he might be taking by opening up and showing vulnerability? The doctor made a note to call Mr. Mason and check in on him.

While documenting the visit and perusing the chart later that afternoon, the doctor made an interesting observation: Although Mr. Mason tried to intimidate, it wasn't clear that he had ever hurt anyone. Three long-term relationships with women played themselves out in the medical record over the span of two decades. Two women who had come to appointments with him were apparently married to Mr. Mason for a few years. There was mention of his putting his hands around their necks or, in one case, threatening to light his wife on fire while she slept, but Mr. Mason was the one who told these stories. Could this be part of a persona he wanted to portray? It was documented that he had been victimized multiple times, including suffering stab wounds. It was possible that Mr. Mason instigated violence, but it was also possible that he just wanted it to appear that way. One of the notes from a medical visit years earlier stated that he denied a charge that landed him in jail—a burglary that he said he did not commit—but he also readily acknowledged that he had committed an earlier offense when he was younger.

A week later, the doctor called Mr. Mason at his new apartment to see how he was doing. It was not a good cell connection, but Mr. Mason sounded pleased to hear from him. Mr. Mason said he had gotten some bedding and winter clothing, but he was not convinced it was clean, so he had soaked it in his tub. He still needed a good pair of boots because there had been snow. He could not stay on the phone long as he said he had to get back to watching several kids. There were children's voices in the background. They ended the call. Mr. Mason never brought up a request for opioids.

The doctor felt he had accomplished what he wanted from the call. He'd engaged in the mundane particulars of Mr. Mason's life, a window into a world far from his own. In so doing, he had shown an interest that he thought might be therapeutic and trust-building. He was playing a long game with his patient through a strategy of asserting clear boundaries combined with persistent respect and caring. He thought he might be able to replace his patient's expectation that doctors can't be trusted and are mainly good for getting pills with something different. He sensed that Mr. Mason craved intimacy and, based on his love for his grandchildren, was capable of it. Although he felt he had made some progress, he also realized that the outbursts directed at him might continue and could be a test of his emotional trustworthiness.

At the same time, the doctor had no illusions that his approach was sure to work. Mr. Mason might be past the point of trusting a doctor—especially a white one. The doctor understood his role and responsibility, which was try to the best of his ability to support a man who had been through much more than he could ever imagine.

How are we to assess the physician's response to patient context described in this case? 4C does not seem adequate to the task. The patient context, here, is the emotional state and temperament of a man who has experienced much trauma in his life and has not been interacting constructively with his care provider. First, consider the contextual probe. Rather than a direct approach, such as "I've noticed you have been angry. Can you tell me why?," which would have been predictably unproductive, the clinician asked, "Can you tell me about the pain you are having?" The clinician appreciated the importance of meeting the patient where he at. Nevertheless, the question still precipitated an outburst which required some give-and-take before the clinician framed it again, this time as "Show me where it's hurting," while coming closer. This physical proximity was also meant to build trust with the patient.

The physician's approach to relationship-building played out over time. Currently, 4C is an effective measure of interactions during a single encounter. 4C does not capture longitudinal interactions with patients. Establishing trust is a dynamic process, meaning that the physician is responding to patient behaviors across and between visits that they cannot predict, and the extent to which that response is attentive to context is key to the success (or lack thereof) of the relationship.

The clinician learned through trial and error an approach to breaking a dysfunctional cycle characterized by conflict during clinical interactions. Setting boundaries demonstrated to Mr. Mason, in a respectful way, that bullying will not get him what he wants (opioids) or alienate his physician (something the physician suspects the patient expects). The physician is direct, unperturbable, caring, and resistant to pressure, creating a safe space for Mr. Mason to open up.

Strong emotions, attitudes, and perspectives form the context for many clinical interactions. And although a physician's response can deeply impact a patient's care, assessing the extent to which it represents a contextualized response is beyond what 4C measures. Part of the problem is simply one of the complexities of a provider's behavior, both verbal and non-verbal. Compare, for instance, a scenario in which a patient has stopped taking a vital medication because of competing responsibilities versus a lack of trust in its safety and effectiveness after the recent death of friend following a serious drug reaction. The former requires some practical problem-solving with the patient to figure out how to get their care plan back on track. The latter requires eliciting and responding therapeutically to a mix of grief, anger, distrust, and fear. It is much more challenging to code for that kind of response.

Although beyond the scope of this chapter, one of us (S. J. W.) recently published a book that explores in depth the interpersonal characteristics of physicians who effectively utilize themselves in patient care.[2] The book posits that physicians who function as healers exhibit two integral personal characteristics in patient interactions: full and open engagement and boundary clarity. A capacity to engage refers to a readiness to connect with others, even across vast differences in life experience. Engagement requires a high degree of personal openness, pleasure in getting to know other people, a lack of fear in the setting of strong emotion, and a feeling of kinship toward others. Boundary clarity enables emotional self-regulation in situations of conflict. It's called "boundary clarity" because it refers to a capacity to distinguish self from other even when emotions are high.

In the care of Mr. Mason, the physician exhibits both. He enters the relationship ready to engage. In the face of the patient's initially hostile response, the physician may have experienced an urge to react but was able distinguish between the patient's behavior and their own emotional response to that behavior, exhibiting boundary clarity. Reflecting on the patient's pattern of interaction with prior physicians, the physician thought about the anxiety and pain these outbursts might serve to disguise. He was able to think about his patient reflectively because he hadn't taken their behavior personally.

4C coders would have given credit to the physician for his response to Mr. Mason's emotional state. But they might also have given credit to the prior physician whose interactions were followed by a fracturing of the relationship. Perhaps because 4C is designed around the principle of "benefit of the doubt," in which coders err on the side of counting any physician response favorably, it may give credit too readily for physician behaviors that fall short of forging connection with a patient in a troubled state. Engaging with boundary clarity is, in our minds, the foundation for a healing interaction. It enables the physician to feel some sense of attachment to their patient, to care *about* them without become enmeshed. The doctor's questions in our example show that he is trying to figure out how he can be most helpful, undistracted by his patient's disruptive behavior. It is conceivable that 4C coders could one day be trained to assess physician engagement and boundary clarity as a response to patients presenting with contextual factors, particularly in domains 7 through 12. In the meantime, we're confident—if without measurement or proof—that showing patients that you care about them through thick and thin is good medicine in any context.

KEY POINTS

- 4C is not well suited to assessing whether a care plan has been contextualized when an appropriate response to patient context is defined by a clinician's interpersonal interactions—such as whether they are open to engage and can maintain boundary clarity.
- The concepts of engagement and boundary clarity are briefly described and illustrated in an extended case. *On Becoming a Healer: The Journey from Patient Care to Caring about Your Patient* explores them in depth and argues that they are essential characteristics of highly effective clinicians.

NOTES

1.   Cameron WB. Informal sociology: a casual introduction to sociological thinking. New York: Random House; 1963.
2.   Weiner SJ. On becoming a healer: the journey from patient care to caring about your patients. Baltimore: Johns Hopkins University Press; 2020.

9

Bringing Context Back into Care

Do not study what disease the patient has; study what patient has the disease.
—Sir William Osler *(attrib.)*

What we have observed, as described in the preceding chapters, is that physicians frequently fail to contextualize care. We see high rates of contextual error: Care plans are often poorly adapted to the circumstances and needs of patients. These contextual errors contribute to medication non-adherence, poor control of chronic conditions, unnecessary emergency department visits, and missed appointments, among many other contextual red flags. Conversely, we've seen that when physicians do contextualize care, their patients have a range of better outcomes, the overall costs of care are lower, and visit times are not longer.

Preventing contextual errors falls mostly to physicians and other clinicians who provide direct patient care. This is in contrast to other kinds of medical errors which can be prevented through systems interventions. If a physician, for instance, accidentally orders 10-fold the correct dose of insulin, multiple safeguards can and should be in place to catch the mistake, a framework known as the "Swiss cheese model." The pharmacist who reviews the order should catch it, as should the nurse who administers the medication; and algorithms in the medical records can serve as safeguards. Like a stack of slices of Swiss cheese, the holes rarely align (although they occasionally do) so that if one person or technology does not prevent an error, another likely will. In contrast, if the physician overlooks evidence that the patient is the one making dosing errors because of failing vision or cognitive deficits or severely arthritic fingers, neither the nurse nor the electronic medical records will catch the oversight because they won't know that it occurred. It's up to physicians to figure out what's going on.

Hence, it seems appropriate to conclude that failures to contextualize care represent a clinician competency deficit. To address the deficit, we propose intervening at each point along the trajectory of the physician's training, starting during the pre-clinical years of medical school and extending through ongoing professional development. In addition, we recognize that medicine is not practiced in a vacuum. Physicians adapt their practice priorities to what is measured and valued when physician performance is assessed. And finally, technology can be a useful aid. Drawing on the findings of studies described in previous chapters, we propose the following strategies.

START EARLY

In recent years medical schools have made a welcome transition from predominantly lecture-based to predominantly case-based approaches to instruction, with an emphasis on active learning. Students are challenged to consider clinical presentations and arrive at evidence-based plans of care. For instance, consider a microbiology class, in which the students must identify an effective antimicrobial therapy for a patient with a multidrug-resistant infectious disease. We would then challenge them to go further: "Okay, now what would you do if you suspected that the patient couldn't afford that medication? What questions would you ask? What would you do if your concerns were confirmed?" We suggest that at least 40% of clinical teaching cases include contextual red flags and factors, to mirror real-world practice.

Such an approach would serve two closely related aims. First, it would be a corrective. The absence of patient context in clinical cases represents a bias in medical training about what types of patient information matter. Second, it would habituate budding clinicians to look for patient context during every medical encounter. They'd arrive at the clinical phase of their training with a broader skill set than most students now have.

Attending to patient life context should be central to how we conceptualize what it means to be a doctor. In fact, the sooner the exposure, the better. Such reframing could begin even before starting medical school. In the United States and Canada, undergraduate education is a pre-requisite for medical training, based on the belief that a liberal arts education is foundational to becoming a physician. Pre-medical requirements currently consist of science and math coursework, plus a varying number of typically unspecified humanities classes. The message is that what's happening inside the body will be critical to patient care but that the interrelationship between body and environment is only vaguely relevant.

Pre-medical teaching could begin with an introduction to the work of George Engel, who introduced the biopsychosocial model.[1] He proposed a hierarchy of interconnected natural systems across a continuum from molecules to biosphere, with the person at the midpoint.[2] Such a framework could be a starting point for examining, at a practical level, how changes to either our bodies or our situation (environment) can disrupt our equilibrium. It would also provide an opportunity to consider how clinicians can help patients re-establish or find a new point of equilibrium. Student aptitude for functioning in such a capacity should be assessed. Everyone who enters medical school should be capable of and interested in seeing others in the context of their life circumstances, past and present. They should have at least an idea of what questions to ask when someone appears emotionally distressed or is behaving in an apparently irrational manner under a range of circumstances and conditions. It is our impression that many who enter medicine do not bring these capabilities.[3] This is not surprising. After all, they are not emphasized during pre-medical training and are not rigorously assessed during the selection process, as far as we are aware. And yet, they are foundational to effective clinical practice.

Currently, pre-medical and medical students are introduced, inconsistently, to a range of ever-shifting social science and humanities concepts that broaden their perspective beyond the biomedical model but lack focus and application. They may be exposed to topics in ethics, psychology, social justice, health policy, international medicine, and so forth. Most recently, the term "social determinants of health" has gained wide currency, and the term "social risk factors" refers to the many stressors that members of marginalized groups experience, including housing instability, food insecurity, and the many adverse health effects of systemic racism and other forms of social injustice. These can be critical patient context. But medicine is a practice, not a body of knowledge. And it is a practice in which the primary instrument is the physician themselves. That instrument needs attention, including calibration and re-calibration. Contextualizing care requires recognizing when a patient may be struggling with life circumstances or self-defeating behaviors, knowing what questions to ask, and then utilizing the information effectively through collaborative dialogue with patients and their families. The process requires self-knowledge because the physician is also a person with emotions, fears, priorities, biases, and insecurities. Without self-knowledge, the physician is a liability during the medical encounter, either detached and task-focused or engaged but often paternalistic, disempowering patients they are supposed to serve and support.

How can we assess whether individuals applying to medical school are interested in caring for patients in the broader context of their life circumstances and will be capable of doing so? It's hard because those who are ambitious learn to say all the right things on their essays and during interviews and volunteer at soup kitchens to bolster their résumés. But at least we can balance what they are expected to learn so that it isn't so lopsided. Currently, getting accepted to medical school requires expending enormous energy excelling in highly demanding science courses such as organic chemistry and biochemistry and then performing well on the Medical College Admissions Test. We are personally skeptical that the depth of the material taught in these courses is warranted. Is it necessary to learn the Friedel-Crafts acylation reaction or pick the most stable carbocation to practice medicine? In contrast, the capacity to discern from the complexity of another person's life that which is relevant to planning their care, the self-knowledge to recognize internal bias, and an openness to engage with people who are suffering, frightened, angry, or confused are essential.

Developing and assessing these capabilities should be at the center, rather than the periphery, of what we teach to, and look for in, future physicians. The challenges of doing so may seem like impediments but should not be. It's easy to tell whether someone knows a chemical reaction but hard to tell if they know how to respond to a human reaction—so we teach and assess the former. All too often we fall into the trap of measuring that which is straightforward to measure rather than measuring what matters. It is reminiscent of the parable of the man who, upon discovering that his keys are missing while walking home late one evening, searches for them under a streetlamp. A kind neighbor comes along and offers to help but with no luck. Finally, the neighbor asks, "So, where were you when you noticed they were missing?" The man points down the street and says, "over there." The neighbor, looking startled, asks "So, why are we looking for them here?" The man replies, "Because, it's where there's light."

INTEGRATE AND REINFORCE

Medical students are highly susceptible to the hidden curriculum, "the unwritten, unofficial, and often unintended lessons, values, and perspectives that students learn in school."[4] What they are taught during their pre-clinical training goes out the window if it is neither reinforced nor valued and, even more so, if it is devalued. Much of their time, especially early on, is spent on the inpatient units caring for hospitalized patients. A predominant message during those clerkships— particularly from residents, who students look up to and spend the most time with—is to be an efficient task completer. There are so many tasks: patients to work up, orders to put in the electronic health record (EHR), notes to write, pre-rounds in the early morning, followed by rounds where they present their patients to an attending, and countless requests from nurses and other staff, calls from families, forms to fill out, and so on. Residents run the show but are likely to value and highly rate those students who help them. On top of that, students must study for their end-of-clerkship exam, which is multiple-choice and has a huge impact on their grade.

Although it is still possible to contextualize care while there are many tasks to complete, it's not foremost on the minds of the care team. From the standpoint of a senior resident running an inpatient service under the supervision of an attending, a priority is keeping the service at a manageable size. This means discharging patients at least at the same rate at which they are admitted. The size of the team managing patients is fixed, so with more patients comes more work for everyone, which can rapidly overwhelm. Furthermore, contextualizing care may be regarded as someone else's responsibility, outsourced to social workers and/or case managers who plan patient discharge.

Undoubtedly, some discharge planners are highly effective. They serve as a bridge between health systems and the patient–family unit, gathering data from the former on a patient's medical and supportive needs and the latter on their support system's capacity to meet those needs. Then, drawing on their knowledge of available community resources and the patient's preferences, they contextualize the discharge plan. That's how it should work. But much can go wrong. Firstly, despite the training social workers receive, which is highly focused on life context, they too are susceptible to the pressures and culture of their work environment. And if the clinicians regard patient context as the social worker's purview, rather than theirs, it makes the job more difficult because of a lack of collaboration.

Watching these dynamics unfold is the impressionable medical student, trying to fit in. In an effort to introduce a corrective to the all-consuming task completer mindset, we embedded an educational intervention to teach and promote contextualization of care during clinical training. As described in Chapter 6 and our publications about the intervention, which was conducted as a randomized controlled trial, we taught students in the intervention group contextualization skills and then had them practice by re-interviewing patients they had admitted the previous night—starting with probes of any contextual red flags.[5] As expected, often they discovered that the team's plan for the patient was inadequate. Our hope was that such an approach would show them, firsthand, that the way they are taught to practice, without explicit attention to patient life context, leaves out vital information that is often essential to effective care.

Although the findings of that study were encouraging in terms of skills acquisition—students in the intervention group demonstrably outperformed the control when tested utilizing standardized patients—it didn't prove that students would actually apply what they learned as a matter of practice during actual patient care. Our subsequent study of residents, in which we taught them the same skills using the same curriculum and assessed them both with standardized patients and unannounced standardized patients (USPs), showed that they were not employing what they learned in practice. Taken together, the findings are emblematic of the famous maxim attributed to legendary management consultant Peter Drucker that "culture eats strategy for breakfast."[6]

There is only one thing that can truly change the culture such that physicians begin to take patient context seriously when planning patient care, and that is to make it a part of how quality is measured and reported. Until then, they will regard it as something that is nice to do but—as long as no one is watching—not a priority. And no matter how well budding physicians are trained to contextualize care, they'll get the message that it's not something that counts. The essential role of measurement in defining what matters is captured in Osborne and Gaebler's often-quoted dictum:[7]

> What gets measured gets done
> If you don't measure results, you can't tell success from failure
> If you can't see success, you can't reward it
> If you can't reward success, you're probably rewarding failure
> If you can't see success, you can't learn from it
> If you can't recognize failure, you can't correct it
> If you can demonstrate results, you can win public support.

DIRECTLY OBSERVE CARE

A major obstacle to measuring contextualization of care is that doing so requires directly observed care (DOC), which itself requires a culture change to implement widely, one more likely to be spurred by a mandate from an external regulatory agency. As we've described in previous chapters, USPs and patient-collected audio are viable and complementary options. Experience has taught us, however, that no matter how strong the evidence that DOC improves patient care and is cost-effective, adoption is unlikely to occur without external pressure. We believe this because the case for DOC is so apparent that the puzzling question is why it's not commonplace already.

The need for DOC goes way beyond assessing contextualization of care.[8] Consider the oddity of spending $4.1 trillion on something annually without directly observing it. Health-care professionals and the quality of their care are assessed indirectly, based on data collected from the medical record and surveys patients fill out about their experience. The actual delivery of care—what happens when the door is closed to the exam room—remains a black box. To consider the status quo acceptable, one would have to believe that not much of import is happening in there that doesn't end up in the medical record or in patient ratings. Furthermore, one would also need to be convinced that the medical record is accurate. And, finally, one would have to be so confident of both as to believe there is no point even checking.

Researchers, including our team, have actually been checking; and there is considerable evidence that the medical record is neither accurate nor complete. In one study, we compared what physicians had written in their note to what our USPs had portrayed as well as audio-recorded during the actual encounter. Across 105 encounters with 36 physicians, there were 636 documentation errors, including 181 errors of commission, in which a clinician documented information that was never elicited (e.g., "patient denies headache or photophobia"), and 455 errors of omission, in which the clinician failed to document clinically significant information (e.g., that penicillin causes "a blotchy itchy rash all the time").[9] Others have found similar problems, including many instances of physicians documenting physical exams that they did not do.[10]

The medical record is particularly poor at capturing variations in meaningful clinician behaviors. For instance, two doctors may both report that they counsel patients to quit smoking when, in fact, one just tells them "You should quit!," whereas the other implements an evidence-based strategy that includes assessing their readiness to quit, recommending tobacco cessation medications, providing a handout of behavioral strategies that help, and scheduling phone follow. We saw such differences in how clinicians approach not only tobacco cessation but also chronic low back pain and depression screening in the USP study we conducted at practices across New Jersey (see Chapter 7).[11] And we were just scratching the surface of assessing the quality of clinician–patient interactions. In virtually every USP study, researchers have found clinically significant deficits in care that are currently undetected. For instance, one USP study demonstrated that a third of primary care physicians provided no skin protective counseling or even recommendations to use a sunscreen during a pre-work physical to lifeguards working on beaches,[12] while another found that 40% of rheumatologists missed the diagnosis of psoriatic arthritis (in USPs with actual psoriatic arthritis) because of a failure to examine their patient's skin.[13] We described these and other studies in a review we published in which we advocated for DOC.[14]

Given our years of experience employing DOC to assess and measurably improve care, we've thought that if anyone has a shot at convincing stakeholders that it's important and they should try it, we might. So we founded the Institute for Practice and Provider Performance Improvement (I3PI) to conduct DOC assessments and interventions to improve health care quality and clinician performance for health-care systems and practices. While we've been hired as consultants on various projects by companies in the health care space, or funded by not-for-profits and even the NIH to study our own innovations, we've had little success with provider organizations specifically to directly observe their care. Conversations with private payers, public payers (Medicare, Medicaid), and health systems leaders are more similar than different. They are fascinated by the concept of DOC, impressed by the data, but not ready to enlist our services. It's evidently not about the money. Even when the Robert Wood Johnson Foundation agreed to pay all the costs, it took a while to find a payer that was game for trying out our USP program.[15]

We've also had limited success at growing the Preventing Contextual Errors program in the Department of Veterans Affairs (VA), despite showing that it prevents hospitalizations, using the VA's own data, and has a return on investment of 75 to 1, as described in Chapter 7.[16] A number of VA leaders are enthusiastic about the program, at both the regional and national levels; but few are ready to invest, despite the evidence. One notable exception is our own facility, where the program has been active since 2012.

It is our impression that the primary impediment to disseminating interventions to prevent contextual error is their reliance on DOC. DOC, put simply, is threatening, particularly to providers and payers. On occasion, in moments of candor, we've heard various versions of "Why would I want someone to come in and expose all kinds of quality problems that are now securely under the rug?" The answer, of course, is because it could help clinicians provide better care to patients. But the asking of the question itself reveals a lot about who has power in health care and who doesn't. Patients are weak players in the marketplace because they have little control over what doctors and hospitals are paid. Contrast this with hospitality and retail, industries where the consumer is king—and which widely employ secret shoppers for direct observation of employee performance.

USE TECHNOLOGY

The EHR is no longer just a platform for documenting and storing patient care-related information. It provides clinical decision support (CDS), alerting clinicians when they might be about to make a mistake and reminding them of things they should probably do, such as recommend preventive care. In addition, EHRs now have patient-facing applications, called "patient portals," that allow patients not only to look at their medical record but also to communicate back to their health-care team and physician. Combining these two features—CDS and the patient interface—is a novel strategy for enabling patients to help their doctors contextualize care. As described in Chapter 7, we've worked with two large EHR systems to develop and test CDS tools that do just that. Our design has two features: a questionnaire the patient completes in the portal and a set of algorithms for automated extraction of contextual red flags from each patient just prior to their visit (e.g., frequent missed appointments, loss of control of a chronic condition). Both drive CDS tools that alert physicians to contextual red flags and factors and guide them to resources or prompt meaningful conversations. Although the technology is certainly not a panacea, it demonstrably helps. Physicians in the intervention arm of the study were more likely to contextualize care.

An advantage of CDS over audit and feedback is that CDS favorably changes clinician behavior in real time. Whereas audit and feedback helps doctors improve their contextualization of care skills going forward, it doesn't benefit the patient who recorded the visit in which the physician made a contextual error. Finally, CDS costs almost nothing to disseminate, in contrast to audit and feedback, which requires an infrastructure for audio-recording visits and analyzing the audio data. None of this is to imply that CDS is better than audit and feedback. Rather, it's complementary and additive. Contextualized CDS should be included as a strategy for increasing contextualization of care.

PUT PATIENTS FIRST (AND DOCTORS WILL BENEFIT TOO)

While exploring how money and power influence health care is beyond our scope, we'd be remiss not to acknowledge their centrality in any discussion about disseminating innovation. Whereas some innovations, such as magnetic resonance imaging (MRI), enhance the status of the profession and bring in new revenue, others, such as DOC, could be perceived to have the opposite effect. These differences, rather than their relative contributions to patient well-being, can drive or suppress their adoption. Whereas MRI provides a window into the patient's body, DOC provides a window into the doctor's exam room. That's a tougher sell because of concerns by powerful stakeholders about what it may reveal.

That said, changes do occur in health care that are initially resisted by doctors but good for patients. For instance, OpenNotes is an international movement that emphasizes transparency between patients and clinicians, to include sharing of the medical record. It took, however, nearly 50 years from the publication of a thought piece in the *New England Journal of Medicine* in 1973, titled "Giving Every Patient His Medical Record: A Proposal to Improve the System," to the passage of the 21st Century Cure Act, which mandates electronic note sharing at no cost.[17]

The expectation that quality is defined by what physicians do during a medical encounter as much as by what they put in the medical record may be coming, but there should be more urgency. Until that day, the doctor–computer relationship will threaten the doctor–patient relationship during the medical encounter, relegating patients to a data source. Our coding team, which listens to thousands of covertly collected recordings of these encounters, comments on the melancholy of hearing countless visits in which the clicking of a keyboard is predominant, as a provider asks lists of questions while entering data into the electronic medical record, and a patient responds passively. As long as the note but not the visit itself counts, the pressure on clinicians is to operate as efficient task completers, rather than as professionals providing whole-person care.

Although innovations are often threatening, they can be a win–win. OpenNotes, resisted so long by providers, is now seen as mutually beneficial. Physicians appreciate that patients have a better understanding of their care and care plan, and some organizations report a decrease in patient e-mails with questions. DOC also has mutual benefits as it recognizes physicians who practice medicine the way so many thought they would when they dreamed of entering the profession. Who goes to medical school because they aspire to sit at a desk and do extensive data entry all day with relatively little human engagement with patients? It's a recipe for burnout, which now affects more than half of physicians in practice. Some may even experience moral injury or, at least, guilt as they sense that they aren't doing what their patients really need.

The future of contextualizing care is tied to the future of DOC. Many physicians will stay trapped in efficient-task-completer mode until they feel recognized rather than penalized for turning away from their computer to face the patient and focus on the most important question at every medical encounter: What is the best next thing for *this* patient at *this* time?

KEY POINTS

- In contrast to other types of medical errors, which are averted by embedding layers of safeguards in systems, contextual errors are averted only by changing the behavior of the people who make them.
- Overcoming a culture that emphasizes efficient task completion over attention to patient life context is a major challenge. Improving physician performance at contextualizing care will require a developmental approach, utilizing different strategies at the pre-clinical and clinical stages of training and during the practice phases of a physician's career. The authors' recommendations include the following:
  - ➤ Starting at the pre-medical phase, provide students with extensive exposure to the biopsychosocial model, with challenging problems to solve in the care of simulated or hypothetical patients with a range of contextual factors. Include examples in which learners must analyze their own emotions and demonstrate a capacity to engage through

role play. There is an urgent need for innovation in substantively and objectively assessing these capabilities during the medical school admissions process and weighting the findings heavily in selection decisions.

➢ In medical school, at the pre-clinical level, embed patient context in case-based learning activities, including team-based learning and problem-based learning, to habituate students to look for contextual red flags and address contextual factors as a routine part of clinical practice.

➢ At both the pre-clinical and clinical phases, provide opportunities to build skills and assess learning with standardized patient cases embedded with patient context.

➢ Meaningful change in how physicians practice will require changing what is measured in performance assessment to include performance at contextualizing care. That will require DOC utilizing patient-collected audio, USPs, or other methods.

➢ Enhance CDS with tools that help clinicians identify and address contextual factors in care planning during the medical encounter.

• Many physicians will feel trapped in efficient-task-completer mode until they no longer feel penalized for turning away from their computer to face the patient and focus on the most important question at every medical encounter: What is the best next thing for *this* patient at *this* time?

NOTES

1. Engel GL. The need for a new medical model: a challenge for biomedicine. Science. 1977;196(4286):129–136.
2. Engel GL. The clinical application of the biopsychosocial model. Am J Psychiatry. 1980;137(5):535–544.
3. Weiner SJ. On becoming a healer: the journey from patient care to caring about your patients. Baltimore: Johns Hopkins University Press; 2020.
4. "Hidden curriculum." The Glossary of Education Reform. Great Schools Partnership. https://www.edglossary.org/hidden-curriculum/. Last accessed July 24, 2022.
5. Schwartz A, Weiner SJ, Harris IB, Binns-Calvey A. An educational intervention for contextualizing patient care and medical students' abilities to probe for contextual issues in simulated patients. JAMA. 2010;304(11):1191–1197.
6. Campbell D, Edgar D, Stonehouse G. Business strategy: an introduction, 3rd ed. London: Palgrave Macmillan; 2011, p. 263.
7. Osborne D, Gaebler T. Reinventing government: how the entrepreneurial spirit is transforming the public sector. Reading, MA: Addison-Wesley Pub. Co.; 1992.
8. Kelley AT, Weiner SJ, Francis J. Directly observed care: crossing the chasm of quality measurement. J Gen Intern Med. 2023;38(1):203–207.
9. Weiner SJ, Wang S, Kelly B, Sharma G, Schwartz A. How accurate is the medical record? A comparison of the physician's note with a concealed audio recording

in unannounced standardized patient encounters. J Am Med Inform Assoc. 2020;27(5):770–775.

10. Dresselhaus TR, Luck J, Peabody JW. The ethical problem of false positives: a prospective evaluation of physician reporting in the medical record. J Med Ethics. 2002;28(5):291–294.

11. Schwartz A, Peskin S, Spiro A, Weiner SJ. Impact of unannounced standardized patient audit and feedback on care, documentation, and costs: an experiment and claims analysis. J Gen Intern Med. 2021;36(1):27–34.

12. Hornung RL, Hansen LA, Sharp LK, Poorsattar SP, Lipsky MS. Skin cancer prevention in the primary care setting: assessment using a standardized patient. Pediatr Dermatol. 2007;24(2):108–112.

13. Gorter S, van der Heijde DM, van der Linden S, et al. Psoriatic arthritis: performance of rheumatologists in daily practice. Ann Rheum Dis. 2002;61(3):219–224.

14. Weiner SJ, Schwartz A. Directly observed care: can unannounced standardized patients address a gap in performance measurement? J Gen Intern Med. 2014;29(8):1183–1187.

15. Schwartz A, Peskin S, Spiro A, Weiner SJ. Direct observation of depression screening: identifying diagnostic error and improving accuracy through unannounced standardized patients. Diagnosis. 2020;7(3):251–256.

16. Weiner S, Schwartz A, Altman L, et al. Evaluation of a patient-collected audio audit and feedback quality improvement program on clinician attention to patient life context and health care costs in the Veterans Affairs health care system. JAMA Netw Open. 2020;3(7):e209644.

17. "Our history: fifty years in the making." OpenNotes. Beth Israel Deaconess Medical Center and Harvard Medical School. https://www.opennotes.org/history/. Last accessed July 24, 2022.

ACKNOWLEDGMENTS

The research and quality improvement activities that we review in this book occurred over nearly two decades of work with many outstanding people. We are particularly indebted to our research team and collaborators. They play keys roles in many chapters, but their intelligence, diligence, and creativity go well beyond what we've been able to capture here.

We commend the medical students, residents, clinical staff, and physicians who have participated in a wide range of projects at the University of Illinois Chicago, in the Veterans Administration (VA) system, and around the Midwest described in *Listening for What Matters*. These dedicated professionals not only agreed to allow themselves to be observed and recorded doing their work but in most cases embraced it as part of their goal to continually improve the care and health of their patients. We are heartened by their trust and commitment. This work would also be impossible without the help of our standardized patient actors and of real patients, particularly veterans, who have carried audio recorders, often concealed, into their visits. Much of the research was supported by the Department of Veterans Affairs, Veterans Health Administration, Office of Research and Development, Health Services Research & Development. Funds for the quality improvement programs are from the Veterans Integrated Service Network 12 and from the Jesse Brown VA Medical Center. Additional support came from the National Board of Medical Examiners' Edward J. Stemmler, MD, Medical Education Research Fund grant, the Robert Wood Johnson Foundation, and the Agency for Healthcare Research and Quality. The views expressed in this book do not necessarily reflect the position or policy of any of the funders, including the Department of Veterans Affairs and the US government.

Amy Binns-Calvey provided valuable feedback on both the first and second editions, for which we are extremely grateful. Craig Panner, our editor at Oxford University Press, was very helpful in shaping the book and helping us work through how best to tell these stories. Of course, any errors or omissions are ours alone. A special debt of gratitude goes to the late Simon Auster, an extraordinary source of insight and guidance from the inception of this work.

We consider this some of our most important work, and we've been supported throughout by some profoundly important people: Suzanne Griffel, Karen Weiner, M. G. Bertulfo, and Ari Schwartz. No words of thanks would be enough.

S. J. W. and A. S.
Chicago, April 2023

BIBLIOGRAPHY

Ball SL, Weiner SJ, Schwartz A, et al. Implementation of a patient-collected audio recording audit & feedback quality improvement program to prevent contextual error: stakeholder perspective. BMC Health Serv Res. 2021;21(1):891.

Bazeley P. (2013). Qualitative data analysis with NVivo (2nd ed.). Thousand Oaks, CA: Sage Publications.

Berwick D. What patient-centered should mean: confessions of an extremist. Health Aff. 2009;28(4):w555–w565. Accessed March 25, 2011. https://www.healthaffairs.org/doi/10.1377/hlthaff.28.4.w555.

Binns-Calvey AE, Malhiot A, Kostovich CT, et al. Validating domains of contextual factors essential to preventing contextual errors: a qualitative study conducted at Chicago area Veterans Health Administration sites. Acad Med. 2017;92(9):1287–1293.

Binns-Calvey AE, Sharma G, Ashley N, Kelley B, Weaver FM, Weiner SJ. Listening to the patient: a typology of contextual red flags in disease management encounters. J Patient Cent Res Rev. 2020;7(1):39–46.

Block L, Habicht R, Wu AW, et al. In the wake of the 2003 and 2011 duty hours regulations, how do internal medicine interns spend their time? J Gen Intern Med. 2013;28(8):1042–1047.

Bloom BS. (1956). Taxonomy of educational objectives: the classification of educational goals (1st ed.). New York: Longmans, Green.

Cameron WB. (1963). Informal sociology: a casual introduction to sociological thinking. New York: Random House.

Dresselhaus TR, Luck J, Peabody JW. The ethical problem of false positives: a prospective evaluation of physician reporting in the medical record. J Med Ethics. 2002;28(5):291–294.

Eccles MP, Mittman BS. Welcome to *Implementation Science*. Implement Sci. 2006;1(1):1.

Engel GL. The clinical application of the biopsychosocial model. Am J Psychiatry. 1980;137(5):535–544.

Engel GL. The need for a new medical model: a challenge for biomedicine. Science. 1977;196(4286):129–136.

Gawande A. (2010). The checklist manifesto: how to get things right (1st ed.). New York: Metropolitan Books.

Glassman PA, Luck J, O'Gara EM, Peabody JW. Using standardized patients to measure quality: evidence from the literature and a prospective study. Jt Comm J Qual Improv. 2000;26(11):644–653.

Gorter S, van der Heijde DM, van der Linden S, et al. Psoriatic arthritis: performance of rheumatologists in daily practice. Ann Rheum Dis. 2002;61(3):219–224.

Graber ML, Franklin N, Gordon R. Diagnostic error in internal medicine. Arch Intern Med. 2005;165:1493–1499.

Graham J. (2010, July 19). Mystery patients' help uncover medical errors. Chicago Tribune.

Green AR, Carney DR, Pallin DJ, et al. Implicit bias among physicians and its prediction of thrombolysis decisions for black and white patients. J Gen Intern Med. 2007;22(9):1231–1238.

Hornung RL, Hansen LA, Sharp LK, Poorsattar SP, Lipsky MS. Skin cancer prevention in the primary care setting: assessment using a standardized patient. Pediatr Dermatol. 2007;24(2):108–112.

Ivers N, Jamtvedt G, Flottorp S, et al. Audit and feedback: effects on professional practice and healthcare outcomes. Cochrane Database Syst Rev. 2012;(6):CD000259. DOI: 10.1002/14651858.CD000259.pub3.

Kelley AT, Weiner SJ, Francis J. Directly observed care: crossing the chasm of quality measurement. J Gen Intern Med. 2023;38(1):203–207.

Kohn LT, Corrigan JM, Donaldson MS, eds. (2000). To err is human: building a safer health system. Washington, DC: National Academies Press.

LaCombe MA. Contextual errors. Ann Intern Med. 2010;153(2):126–127.

Livingstone R. (1946, November). Education for the modern world. The Atlantic, 75–79.

Luck J, Peabody JW. Using standardised patients to measure physicians' practice: validation study using audio recordings. BMJ. 2002;325(7366):679.

Luck J, Peabody JW, Dresselhaus TR, Lee M, Glassman P. How well does chart abstraction measure quality? A prospective comparison of standardized patients with the medical record. Am J Med. 2000;108(8):642–649.

National Academies of Sciences, Engineering, and Medicine. 2019. Integrating social care into the delivery of health care: moving upstream to improve the nation's health. Washington, DC: National Academies Press. https://doi.org/10.17226/25467.

Osborne D, Gaebler T. (1992). Reinventing government: how the entrepreneurial spirit is transforming the public sector. Reading, MA: Addison-Wesley Pub. Co.

Peabody JW, Luck J, Glassman P, Dresselhaus TR, Lee M. Comparison of vignettes, standardized patients, and chart abstraction: a prospective validation study of 3 methods for measuring quality. JAMA. 2000;283(13):1715–1722.

Reason JT. (1990). Human error. Cambridge, England; New York: Cambridge University Press.

Rodwin BA, Bilan VP, Merchant NB, et al. Rate of preventable mortality in hospitalized patients: a systematic review and meta-analysis. J Gen Intern Med. 2020;35(7):2099–2106.

Rosenhan DL. On being sane in insane places. Clin Soc Work J. 1974;2(4):237–256.

Ross L. The intuitive psychologist and his shortcomings: distortions in the attribution process. Adv Exp Social Psychol. 1977;10:173–220.

Roter D, Larson S. The Roter interaction analysis system (RIAS): utility and flexibility for analysis of medical interactions. Patient Educ Couns. 2002;46(4):243–251. DOI: 10.1016/s0738-3991(02)00012-5.

Schwartz A. Toward a patient right to record medical visits. UIC Law Rev. 2023;57(1).

Schwartz A, Peskin S, Spiro A, Weiner SJ. Direct observation of depression screening: identifying diagnostic error and improving accuracy through unannounced standardized patients. Diagnosis. 2020;7(3):251–256.

Schwartz A, Peskin S, Spiro A, Weiner SJ. Impact of unannounced standardized patient audit and feedback on care, documentation, and costs: an experiment and claims analysis. J Gen Intern Med. 2021;36(1):27–34.

Schwartz A, Weiner SJ, Binns-Calvey A, Weaver FM. Providers contextualise care more often when they discover patient context by asking: meta-analysis of three primary data sets. BMJ Qual Saf. 2016;25(3):159–163.

Schwartz A, Weiner SJ, Harris IB, Binns-Calvey A. An educational intervention for contextualizing patient care and medical students' abilities to probe for contextual issues in simulated patients. JAMA. 2010;304(11):1191–1197.

Schwartz A, Weiner SJ, Weaver F, et al. Uncharted territory: measuring costs of diagnostic errors outside the medical record. BMJ Qual Saf. 2012;21(11):918–924.

Sutton RT, Pincock D, Baumgart DC, Sadowski DC, Fedorak RN, Kroeker KI. An overview of clinical decision support systems: benefits, risks, and strategies for success. NPJ Digit Med. 2020;3:17.

Weiner S, Schwartz A, Altman L, et al. Evaluation of a patient-collected audio audit and feedback quality improvement program on clinician attention to patient life context and health care costs in the Veterans Affairs health care system. JAMA Netw Open. 2020;3(7):e209644.

Weiner SJ. Contextualizing care: fireside chat series. YouTube, February 6, 2022. https://youtube.com/playlist?list=PL9-b6XZZMupzmVuuwn1Ipph0dpI1fxx2d. Last accessed May 25, 2022.

Weiner SJ. Contextualizing medical decisions to individualize care: lessons from the qualitative sciences. J Gen Intern Med. 2004;19(3):281–285.

Weiner SJ. From research evidence to context: the challenge of individualizing care. ACP J Club. 2004;141(3):A11–A12.

Weiner SJ. (2020). On becoming a healer: the journey from patient care to caring about your patients. Baltimore: Johns Hopkins University Press.

Weiner SJ. When "something is missing" from the resident's presentation. Acad Med. 2004;79(1):101.

Weiner SJ, Ashley N, Binns-Calvey A, Kelly B, Sharma G, Schwartz A. Content coding for contextualization of care. Version 13.0, Released May 27, 2021. Harvard Dataverse Network Project. https://dataverse.harvard.edu/dataverse/4C.

Weiner SJ, Kelly B, Ashley N, et al. Content coding for contextualization of care: evaluating physician performance at patient-centered decision making. Med Decis Making. 2014;34(1):97–106.

Weiner SJ, Schwartz A. Directly observed care: can unannounced standardized patients address a gap in performance measurement? J Gen Intern Med. 2014;29(8):1183–1187.

Weiner SJ, Schwartz A, Sharma G, et al. Patient-centered decision making and health care outcomes: an observational study. Ann Intern Med. 2013;158(8):573–579.

Weiner SJ, Schwartz A, Sharma G, et al. Patient-collected audio for performance assessment of the clinical encounter. Jt Comm J Qual Patient Saf. 2015;41(6):273–278.

Weiner SJ, Schwartz A, Weaver F, et al. Contextual errors and failures in individualizing patient care: a multicenter study. Ann Intern Med. 2010;153(2):69–75.

Weiner SJ, Schwartz A, Weaver F, et al. Effect of electronic health record clinical decision
    support on contextualization of care: a randomized clinical trial. JAMA Netw Open.
    2022;5(10):e2238231.

Weiner SJ, Wang S, Kelly B, Sharma G, Schwartz A. How accurate is the medical re-
    cord? A comparison of the physician's note with a concealed audio recording
    in unannounced standardized patient encounters. J Am Med Inform Assoc.
    2020;27(5):770–775.

Saul J. Weiner, MD, at Jesse Brown VA Medical Center and the University of Illinois at Chicago College of Medicine (UIC COM), and **Alan Schwartz, PhD**, UIC COM, have spent the last twenty years studying physicians' attention to patient life context during the medical encounter. Their work, involving undercover actors and real patients carrying concealed audio recorders, has been published in *Annals of Internal Medicine, JAMA—The Journal of the American Medical Association, BMJ Quality & Safety, The Joint Commission Journal of Quality and Patient Safety, Medical Decision Making*, and many other publications. They are also the founders and principals of the Institute for Practice and Provider Performance Improvement (I3PI), a public benefit corporation that brings these techniques from research into practice.

For the benefit of digital users, indexed terms that span two pages (e.g., 52–53) may, on occasion, appear on only one of those pages.

Tables and figures are indicated by *t* and *f* following the page number